Managing Managed Care

Managing Managed Care

Psychotherapy and Medication Management in the Modern Era

Robert Langs

JASON ARONSON

Lanham • Boulder • New York • Toronto • Plymouth, UK

Published in the United States of America
by Jason Aronson
An imprint of Rowman & Littlefield Publishers, Inc.

A wholly owned subsidiary of
The Rowman & Littlefield Publishing Group, Inc.
4501 Forbes Boulevard, Suite 200, Lanham, Maryland 20706
www.rowmanlittlefield.com

Estover Road
Plymouth PL6 7PY
United Kingdom

British Library Cataloguing in Publication Information Available

Library of Congress Cataloging-in-Publication Data

Langs, Robert, 1928–
Managing managed care : psychotherapy and medication management in the modern era / Robert Langs.
p. ; cm.
Includes bibliographical references and index.
ISBN-13: 978-0-7657-0576-1 (cloth : alk. paper)
eISBN-13: 978-0-7657-0651-5
1. Managed mental health care. I. Title.
[DNLM: 1. Psychotherapy—organization & administration. 2. Managed Care Programs—economics. WM 460 L285m 2009]
RC465.6.L36 2009
362.2'0425—dc22 2008047649

Printed in the United States of America

™ The paper used in this publication meets the minimum requirements of American National Standard for Information Sciences—Permanence of Paper for Printed Library Materials, ANSI/NISO Z39.48-1992.

Contents

Preface

Scenes from managed care practices:

A male therapist is seeing a woman patient in managed care psychotherapy. He files an outpatient treatment request to the insurer for fifteen additional sessions. The request is lost by the insurer and both the patient and the therapist receive notice that the patient's sessions are no longer authorized. The therapist then files a new request form and the insurer responds by asking the therapist to provide copies of his process notes on the therapy and to complete a detailed questionnaire, four pages long, on the course and status of the treatment. After discussing it with the patient and obtaining her approval, the therapist complies. Two weeks later, the insurer approves ten more sessions for the patient. That week, the patient telephones the therapist and abruptly quits treatment.

In another situation, an insurer fails to pay a bill submitted by a woman therapist for a consultation session with a depressed female patient; no reason is given. The therapist investigates the problem and is told that while this insurer covers the patient for medical services, another insurer covers the patient for psychotherapy. The therapist submits a bill to the second insurer but it is returned to her because they require prior authorization for psychotherapy sessions and none had been requested. The therapist inquires further and is told that it is too late for the insurer to back-date the authorization and that she should submit a new bill, wait for it to be rejected, and then file an appeal. She does so and two months later the appeal is approved and she is paid her fee. Meanwhile, the patient, who has been informed of these transactions, becomes very mistrustful of the therapist and confesses that of late, she has not been telling the therapist everything that had been coming to her mind. The therapy continues, but ends three months later with limited results.

Another woman therapist is treating an adolescent girl who is a dependent of an insured father. The therapist submits a bill that the insurance company fails to pay pending an investigation of the child's status. Months later, after the patient has unexpectedly terminated treatment, the therapist is informed that the child, who had dropped out of school, is not covered by the father's policy. The therapist bills the patient and then her father for the fee set by the insurer, but does not receive payment.

A woman patient calls a male therapist to make an urgent appointment for an evaluation for psychotherapy and the therapist offers her a suitable hour. He explains that he is putting the time aside for her and asks that she take responsibility to keep the appointment. The patient agrees to do so, but without calling the therapist, she does not appear for the session. The therapist bills the patient for the missed session, but to no avail.

Finally, an insurer instructs a psychotherapist-provider to have his patient sign a release that allows the therapist to send confidential information about the patient's psychotherapy to his primary care physician. When the form is presented to the patient, he tells the therapist that his primary care physician has a big mouth and he doesn't trust him with this kind of information. Besides, he adds, he sees him once a year for a physical examination and they never discuss the patient's personal life. He refuses to sign the form and soon begins to be late for, and more resistant during, his sessions.

Endless themes and variations, many of them with unexpected twists that confound and distress both patient and therapist, incidents that have discouraged both beneficiaries and potential providers from engaging in psychotherapy or medication management under the auspices of managed care insurers. Overlooked in the midst of these somewhat daunting incidents and the chaos they cause is the fact that many of these potentially harmful situations can be avoided and if inescapable, can be dealt with effectively and made to serve the emotion-related healing of the patient. Managed care psychotherapy and medication management can and should be viable and effective undertakings that are, all in all, highly rewarding experiences for all concerned—patient, therapist, and insurer. But for this to happen, the therapeutic work needs to be grounded in a sound set of basic insights and in effective therapeutic principles of the kind to be offered in this book.

In this regard, notice that every one of these representative problems has little or nothing to do with how a therapist does psychotherapy—incidents of this kind come up in the practices of all manner of managed care psychotherapists and psychiatrists. Instead, these issues revolve around the ground rules, boundaries, and framework—the conditions, contractual and otherwise—of the managed care treatment process. Despite beliefs to the contrary, the conditions under which therapy is conducted are not peripheral to the treatment experience and process of cure, but are an essential part of the therapeutic experience and a major factor in its success or failure. Recognizing that this is the case has been problematic mainly because the most telling effects of the therapist's management of the ground rules of therapy—and of the rules themselves—are mediated unconsciously. It follows, then, that no matter how a therapist does therapy, it is essential for him or her to grasp the profound effects of the deep unconscious experiences, frame-related and otherwise, of the human mind. As it turns out, the deep unconscious mind is not only frame-sensitive, it also is frame-wise in that, as an adaptive intelligence, it fully grasps the extensive effects of the ground rules of treatment and has a definitive awareness of the ideal or archetypal frame. As a result, this overlooked system of the mind is a critical resource in managing managed care therapies. Indeed, the outcome of most managed care treatment experiences depends heavily on identifying and following the wise advisories of the deep unconscious mind.

For better or worse, managed care mental health services of one kind or another are now the primary means through which individuals world-wide receive assistance designed to alleviate their emotional suffering and the conflicts and maladaptations on which it is based. Created to deliver effective services to as many individuals as possible, these efforts, which take shape as some form of psychotherapy or counseling with or without psychotropic medications, have had many notable successes. Nevertheless, there also have been significant failures largely because of the many unresolved problems intrinsic to the basic structure of these treatment modalities. Offering the means of resolving as many of these obstacles to cure as possible is another major goal of the present volume.

Of the many factors that determine the outcome of a managed care psychotherapy experience—the nature of the patient's emotional problems, the type of therapy offered by the therapist, the historical background of each, and the conditions under which treatment is offered—the one factor that cuts across all such efforts is the framework of treatment. In this light, we can no longer think simplistically that a therapist can do little more than ply his or her trade under the conditions imposed by managed care insurers—i.e., that these conditions are not crucial matters of concern. Instead, we must realize that the conditions of therapy are as important to the therapeutic process as — and at time more important than—the active therapeutic ministrations offered by a therapist, be they interpretations, cognitive exercises, or whatever. For this reason among many others, the present volume will be focused on the rules, frames, and boundaries of managed care psychotherapies and efforts at medication management. It is thereby offered to therapists of all backgrounds and persuasions.

To conclude this introduction on a more personal note, it is my belief as the founder of a new way of listening to and understanding the human mind and its hidden proclivities, that it was incumbent on me to undertake a fresh investigation of the basic components of the managed care situation. I have worked as a managed care psychiatrist and psychotherapist for nearly ten years now and have been a member of a committee set up by a major insurer to review and respond to complaints made by patients against their mental health providers. I have seen first-hand the constructive efforts that are being made by insurers to try to make available to their insurees the best possible care and have monitored insurers' efforts to be fair to, and responsive to the needs of, their providers as well. But I also have seen many abuses, some of them unthinkable yet blithely enacted—clients exploiting both insurers and their providers; insurers and providers exploiting their patients; and providers deceiving and taking illegal advantage of the insurance companies with whom they have contracted. While the terrible ramifications of these dreadful dramas often do not register consciously in the parties involved, everyone is the loser in these moments of uncalled-for abuse.

I held back from doing managed care psychotherapy for many years because I anticipated a mine-field of problems, most of them frame-related and many of them likely to be beyond repair and detrimental to myself and my patients. My experiences with private psychotherapy had revealed many harmful consequences for all concerned in operating under less than ideal conditions and ground rules for a treatment experience. I was skeptical, then, about my hope to accomplish effective healing under the deviant conditions of managed care therapy. Nevertheless, largely because of financial pressures, I began to do managed care psychotherapy and medication management hoping that I could finds way to lessen the effects of the less-than-ideal frame under which I would be working and thereby be helpful to my patients in some lasting way. I was fully aware that the income so derived would arrive in small, demeaning increments but I also was aware that necessity is the mother of risk—and hope.

Much to my surprise and delight, I proved to be quite mistaken in respect to most of my dire expectations—a striking illustration of the extent to which so-called "conscious thought experiments" in the emotional realm tend to be in error. I had, for example, anticipated that I would have to settle for using an over-intellectualized and extremely limited therapeutic approach, but to the contrary, I found that I could obtain meaningful narratives—encoded dreams and stories—from many of these patients and thus make full use of adaptive therapeutic principles of technique in working with and interpreting their material and insightfully resolving their emotion-related symptoms (Langs 2004, 2006). I also unexpectedly discovered that, with most patients, the mandated departures from the ideal conditions of treatment tended to fade into the background and were not a significant, extended source of resistance or an intractable obstacle to the process of cure.

The resultant sense of hope and promise, which was grounded in deep unconsciously derived insights into the therapeutic process and the role—advantageous and at times, disadvantageous—of the framework of managed care therapy did much to motivate me to write this book. My purpose is manifest and self-evident: To help therapists of all persuasions to enhance their healing efforts under managed care conditions of treatment and to make doing such work optimally satisfying for all concerned—patients, therapists, and their insurers. With this heartfelt goal in mind, I turn now to my clinically grounded studies of the conditions and transactions of managed psychotherapy and medication management, their therapeutic potential, and their most common pitfalls and most viable solutions. In order to provide a solid foundation for this effort, I shall begin by offering some fresh perspectives on the human mind and the psychotherapeutic process through which its maladaptations and dysfunctions may be alleviated.

Robert Langs, M.D.
New York City,
September, 2008

Chapter One

The Mind in Context

It is no longer tenable to approach managed care psychotherapy and medication management solely on the basis of common sense, intuition, and a still uncertain, debatable theoretical orientation. Recent research into both the *mind* and the *brain* that sponsors its activities has shown that mental operations and emotion-related adaptations are quite complex and as such, regardless of how one does psychotherapy, they deserve extensive, in-depth scrutiny, understanding, and application. Success in these efforts will allow us to develop therapeutic principles that can inform and enhance every mode of psychotherapy and psychopharmacology in practice today. The failure to establish universal principles has led to countless errant interventions by mental health professionals that have caused harm to their patients and themselves. With this in mind, I shall set forth a set of basic, clinically derived guidelines that will, in turn, provide us with a solid, supportive structure for the conduct of the managed care treatment modalities that are the subject of this book.

The therapeutic principles that I shall espouse are derived from a group of newly discovered *universal mental archetypes* that are relevant to all modes of emotion-related healing. By and large, these archetypes, which account for the design and preferences of the conscious mind, are not reflected in conscious adaptations, which are far more individualized than universally shared. Thus, the critical archetypes of the emotion processing mind are not to be found in the surface or manifest communications of patients—or their therapists—a finding that accounts for both the general lack of awareness of these basics principles and for the great variety of consciously forged forms of psychotherapy. These archetypes, which involve universally shared perceptions of the meanings of emotion-related events and a set of ideal coping strategies with which to deal with them, are unconsciously wrought and thus, reflected solely in the encoded meanings embedded in the dreams and other storied messages from patients. These deep unconscious perceptions and adaptive responses, which are both universal and optimally adaptive, will serve us well in identifying the most effective ways that managed care therapy can be practiced.

The basic understanding of the human mind and therapeutic interaction that will be presented here involves several inter-related realms of conceptualization. They include the evolved design of the human mind and its main emotion-related subsystem, the so-called *emotion-processing mind*; the resultant psychodynamics of emotional dysfunctions; the conscious and unconscious communications, adaptive activities, and psychodynamic forces that are involved in the process of emotional healing; and lastly, the profound influence of the rules, frames, and boundaries under which such efforts are conducted.

These considerations characterize the *adaptive approach* on which this book is based. This new paradigm of human psychology and adaptation is deeply grounded in the psychobiology of the human mind. While it was forged from clinical observations, it can be derived from and is keeping with the well tested principles of biology in which adaptation and survival are recognized as the basic tasks of all living organisms. The result is a view of the mind as a whole and the specialized module of the mind that has evolved to cope to emotionally charged impingements—the so-called *emotion-processing mind*—as adaptive entities that have evolved to deal with adverse environmental changes and thus psychological and physical traumas. Optimizing the ability of the emotion-processing mind to deal with these traumas, including those that that occur in the course of a patient's psychotherapy experience as well as those that were the source of a patient's emotional ills, stands high among the goals of this book. It is in this regard that the archetypes of sound psychotherapy will prove to be most illuminating and helpful.

Throughout the natural world, that is, for both living and inanimate entities, boundary conditions exert an enormous influence on the transactions that take place within their confines. Information about the status of the boundaries of a system provides an observer with a great deal of vital knowledge about what is happening in its interior. Thus, efforts at emotion-related healing, whatever they may be, cannot be considered in isolation, but must be explored and understood in light of the setting and the ground rules that frame these endeavors. Indeed, the environment established for a psychotherapy experience, the amount of structure and its particular features, greatly affect the moment-to-moment transactions between a patient and his or her therapist.

These frame-related effects depend on a wide range of factors and may at any given moment be positively or negatively cast. Indeed, environmental influences may affect both patients and their therapists by contributing to symptomatic regressions on the one hand and clinical relief on the other. Yet despite its enormous influence, a look at the psychotherapeutic literature indicates that the framework of therapy is seldom if at all subjected to the detailed scrutiny and respectful attention it deserves.

As reported to me by patients with whom I conducted medication consultations, this neglect of the frame is common among all manner of psychotherapists and especially prominent in the practice of managed care medicating psychiatrists. Indications are that medication management is widely practiced without clear basic standards and thus, with a lack of underlying structure and poor to loose boundaries and ground rules—if any. Indications are that as a result, much had gone awry in these efforts at medication management and in the therapeutic efforts of the various types of therapists who referred these patients to me for psychotropic assistance. These patients tended to suffer unduly without a modicum of insight into the ways in which their poorly structured treatments were causing them harm. Paradoxically, most often these patients expressed satisfaction with their therapists or prior psychiatrists even though their symptoms had not been alleviated and in most cases, had intensified. The conscious minds of patients—and of us as their therapists—are extremely unreliable judges of the efficacy and drawbacks of the therapeutic approaches that address emotional difficulties. One reason for this state of affairs is that most of the damaging consequences of unprincipled interventions and poorly managed frameworks of treatment are mediated unconsciously, outside of the awareness of either party to therapy, and in addition, their patently evident existence is blocked out of awareness and denied consciously by both patient and therapist. For this reason, I shall of necessity pay close attention to the unconscious realm of experience and its effects on the patients and therapists who work under managed care conditions.

THE NEGLECT OF GROUND RULES AND FRAMES

Whatever form treatment takes, there are many reasons why the powerful effects of the conditions of therapy have not been afforded the recognition they deserve. The first lies with the way in which therapists of all persuasions listen to and formulate the material from their patients. The focus is on the manifest contents and extractable implications of their patients' material which, despite attempts to formulate meanings of which the patient is unaware, basically is a conscious system effort that precludes the decoding of the critical encoded messages from the deep unconscious mind regarding the treatment experience in general and the prevailing ground rules in particular. This approach is driven by unconscious needs that pertain to therapists' fears of secured frames, an anxiety they unknowingly share with their patients who also prefer superficial approaches to the ground rules in which misguided flexibility is the rule. Managed care therapies have suffered greatly because both parties to therapy tend consciously to ignore the sizable effects of the conditions of treatment and because both have a natural conscious predilection for loosely managed, poorly structured frames that serve to deny death and its attendant anxieties regardless of the cost.

There are two major, inter-related additional underlying factors in this widespread neglect of ground rules and frames. The first lies with the nature of present thinking about the human mind and the emotional difficulties from which it may suffer. Both cognitive and psychodynamic psychologies are mind-centered in that they propose that emotion-related symptoms, both intrapsychic and interpersonal in nature, are primarily the result of disorders of the mind. Environmental and interactional factors are now gaining some attention, but they are viewed as secondary considerations and treated in a broad and indefinite manner that severely limits their relevance and usefulness.

The second additional factor in the neglect of frames lies with the above noted ways in which ground rule conditions and issues activate concerns with death and the three forms of death anxiety that we experience as humans. The conscious mind tends to avoid and obliterate these concerns and everything to which they are attached. In a sense, then, avoiding frames is akin to denying death and denying death is the default position of the conscious mind.

One of the main results of our neglect of the effects of the ground rules of treatment is a widespread failure to recognize the existence of an ideal, archetypal set of ground rules and boundaries that enhances all types of emotion-related healing. The conscious mind, which is strongly geared for defense and the overuse of denial, has no means of recognizing this critical archetype, which is, however, universally recognized and supported by the deep unconscious minds of both patients and their therapists. By and large, then, we cannot turn to the conscious mind to define and clinically fashion an ideal, healing set of ground rules for managed care treatment situations; it is, by design, incapable of doing so. We must turn instead to decoding the disguised messages from the deep unconscious mind for the framework we need to enhance our emotion-related therapeutic efforts. Much as all roads point to Rome, all frame-related needs point to accessing the deep unconscious mind.

BASIC APPROACHES TO PSYCHOTHERAPY

In respect to psychotherapy, there are three basic ways to approach and attempt to alleviate or heal a patient's emotional maladaptations—cognitively, psychodynamically, and psychopharmacologically. With the exception of the adaptive version of psychoanalysis, none of these modes of treatment operate on the basis of established principles for structuring a psychotherapy experience and are grounded in general principles of technique that as yet await clear validation. As for ground rules, in general, the further an approach's distance from a dynamic form of psychotherapy, the greater the likelihood that the framework of treatment will receive little if any thought and that departures from, and violations of, the ideal archetypal framework of treatment will be commonplace.

Cognitive-Behavioral Approaches

Therapists who work using some version of cognitive-behavioral therapy, a broadly defined treatment modality that appears to dominate the present-day therapeutic scene, tend to address and work with the manifest expressions of their patients' emotion-related problems and base their interventions on both their own theoretical orientation and the patients' manifest communications as they describe and address their symptoms. These therapists and counselors are inclined to set aside and to see no need to define and consider the hidden, psychodynamically unconscious factors in emotional disorders and their alleviation.

Cognitive treatment approaches tend to vary, but in principle, they are directed at trying to alter the patient's conscious thinking, feelings, and overt behaviors. Essentially, then, this is a "modify the symptom" approach. This is the spirit behind cognitive retraining, as seen with the attempt to cure a depression by teaching patients how to eradicate their unhappy thoughts and replace them with happy ones. Other cognitive approaches include efforts at deconditioning, advice-giving, hypnotherapy, the offer of emotion-related exercises and tasks, and direct exploratory work with the surface contents of patients' material in order to reframe or recontexturalize the relevant issues. The basic goal is to favorably modify an existing symptom by focusing on the present; little attention is paid to the past relationships and traumas which underlie a current emotion-related problem.

In sum, then, cognitive therapeutic techniques are directed at the conscious mind and its cognitive operations. Most of this work is symptom-focused. It is thereby patient-focused, rather than interactively conceptualized, and centered entirely on conscious mental operations. There is an implicit recognition of unconscious factors, but they are not viewed dynamically. Instead, they are thought of as the hidden forces beneath cognitive patterns and their alteration.

As can be seen, aside from general notions related to stress and trauma, there is little or no place in these approaches for the role played by the conditions under which a symptom has developed. Much the same applies to the framework of the various variants of cognitive treatment. In general, however, when ground rules are touched on, therapists working with these approaches endorse or accept a wide range of departures from the universal archetypal frame that optimizes an emotion-related healing experience. The prevailing position among cognitive therapists is either that the frame is of little or no consequence to the therapeutic experience and treatment outcome or that each therapist is entitled to establish the particular set of ground rules within which he or she prefers to work or seems best for a given patient. This "select the frame you think best" attitude overlooks the existence of a deep unconsciously, universally preferred archetypal frame and fails to recognize that departures from this frame may be extremely harmful to both patients and their therapists. This denial of the existence of frame-related archetypes plays a significant role in the neglect of the frame in all manner of emotion-related therapeutic efforts.

Common examples of these departures from the ideal frame that are often seen in cognitive therapies include a laying on of the hands in which therapists engage in sanctioned physical contact with their patients; the offer of a wide range of opinions and personal self-revelations; the use of non-professional locales including home settings for the therapy; irregular scheduling of sessions; contacts with patients outside of the treatment setting—and much more. Given that the frameworks of managed care therapies are themselves fundamentally far from ideal, the clinical finding that frame modifications tend to beget frame modifications suggests that these departures from the ideal set of ground rules will be more frequent in managed care treatment situations than in private forms of therapy where some semblance of a basic frame may be offered. This is a serious matter because frame violations tend to escalate, often to the point where major damage is done to the patient—and therapist as well. This means that even though they are disinclined to deal with the unconsciously mediated meanings and effects of the ground rule conditions of their therapeutic ministrations, cognitive behavioral therapists are well advised to learn about this aspect of therapy. Doing so will greatly enhance their treatment efforts and spare them much disruptive deep unconscious guilt and unconsciously driven efforts at self-punishment for the therapeutic failures that departures from the archetypal frame tend to cause.

Psychodynamic Approaches

The second basic approach to resolving emotion-related symptoms involves working within a psychodynamic framework in which competing forces, conflict, and to some extent deprivation and trauma are seen to play a role. Despite their commitment to understand and take into account the unconscious aspects of emotional maladaptations and to effect their resolution through psychotherapy, the mode of listening and formulating utilized by analytically-oriented psychotherapists is quite restricted and in turn, its use has limited the range of understanding and the therapeutic techniques used by these therapists.

By and large, the search for unconscious factors carried out in dynamic forms of listening has focused on the implications of patients' manifest messages, especially those implications and seeming early life sources of which the patient is consciously unaware. These extracted meanings are, at most, superficially unconscious in that they are easily detected. Clinically, these formulations of unconscious implications and their postulated links to early childhood experiences tend to be either self-evident or arbitrarily formulated by the therapist and they lack emotional importance and power. There also is no reliable means of validating a therapist's—or patient's—interpretation of the available material. All in all, these efforts tend to be arbitrary, highly intellectualized, theory-driven, and without the anxiety-provoking effects seen when deeply unconscious perceptions and traumas emerge into awareness. The key idea, however, is that a patient's emotional problems primarily are internally driven, with secondary effects from others and the environment. Patients' inner-mental disturbances are variously thought to be caused by errant sexual, interpersonal, narcissistic, or other troublesome needs and wishes. They are thought to find expression in the interaction with the therapist, usually in the form of *transferences*, which reflect a patient's distorted view of his or her therapist based on damaging early life experiences. In general, in the course of a dynamic form of treatment, these transferences and other expressions of emotional pain are examined directly, traced to their early roots in the patient's interactions with his or her parents and significant others, and are said to be resolved insightfully—however superficial this effort may be.

An inner-mental disease concept is basic to the psychotherapy offered by present-day psychodynamically and psychoanalytically oriented psychotherapists. The focus is on the inner wishes and needs of patients as they emerge in the interaction with the therapist. There are several different schools or sub-theories of psychoanalysis that lay claim to the primary needs whose dysfunctions are the root cause of emotional symptoms. They include classical drive theory, which centers on forbidden Oedipal and incestuous wishes towards the parent of the opposite sex; object relations theory, which centers on relational needs; interpersonal and intersubjective theories that focus on interactional needs and wishes; self-psychology, which sees narcissistic needs as the core problem in emotional life; and a handful of other such schools of thought and theory.

These approaches are identified as psychoanalytic because they theorize that unconscious needs and wishes play a significant role in an emotional disorder and the therapeutic process. Empirically, however, these unconscious expressions are arbitrarily understood to involve anything that the patient is unaware of in his or her behaviors, symptoms, or communications. These unrecognized meanings are extracted from the material generated by the patient and they often are self-evident, even though the patient seems to have missed them. For example, these therapists may try to relieve a patient's depression by showing him or her how the implications of their messages reflect dysfunctional patterns of relating, interacting with others, managing their sexual or aggressive drives, taking care of their self-image, and such. In addition, based on the belief that these difficulties have their main sources in a variety of disturbing early childhood experiences between the patient and his or her caretakers and others of importance, these aberrant patterns are traced back to events that took place in these problem-promoting relationships.

All of these efforts are focused on the internal workings of the human mind and pay only minimal, secondary attention to the outer world, that is, to the stimuli that evoke these needs and to the actual conditions under which they are explored in a psychotherapy experience. There is, then, little felt need to explore adaptations to the environment and their role in the etiology of emotional ills and the therapy experience.

As a final perspective, it is well to note that despite his inner-mental focus and failure to recognize the effects modifications of the framework of psychoanalysis, Freud nevertheless was mindful in principle of the importance of the conditions under which a psychoanalysis is conducted. In his early papers on the technique of psychoanalysis, he devoted as much space to the ground rules as he did to the subjects of transference and interpretation. He commented on the need to sustain the analyst's neutrality and anonymity, the importance of confidentiality, and, in a broad manner, he also explored the effects of the fee on the analytic experience. Even so, in practice he worked in an office located in the same building as his living quarters, spoke to patients about his family and other patients, fed some of his patients during their sessions and invited others into his flat for a meal, saw some patients without charging them a fee, allowed patients to trade session times, and published case material using little in the way of disguise. The many unorthodox ways in which he managed the framework of analysis and practiced his trade indicate that one aspect of Freud's genius was that he identified many of the ideal, archetypal ground rules of analysis and psychotherapy even though he himself never made use of them. His self-contradictory and confusing heritage is reflected in the wide range of beliefs and conflicting opinions regarding the framework of psychotherapy that prevails among psychoanalysts today and is partly responsible for their failure to discover and articulate a clear set of basic principles in this regard.

Psychopharmacology

As is well known, psychopharmacologists attempt to positively modify patients' conscious mood states, thinking, and emotionally founded symptoms through the use of psychotropic medications—that is, chemically and psychobiologically. Their main pursuit is the search for the optimal drug, given at the optimal dosage. The vicissitudes of patients' symptoms are tracked and possible side effects are documented. The central decisions involve the level of relief that the patient is experiencing, whether to shift to a new medication if the present offering seems to be failing the patient, the nature of possible side effects and how they should be dealt with, and similar drug-related issues.

This form of treatment is almost entirely symptom- and drug-centered; little or no attention is paid to other matters, including the nature and effects of the ground rules of treatment. In managed care settings, brief sessions are common and there is virtually no opportunity for patients to talk about anything other than medication-related issues. The psychiatrist or nurse practitioner therefore has little chance to hear about ground rule issues even though departures from the ideal frame—for example, the presence of secretaries, variabilities in scheduling to see patients, and the use of hospital- or shared-office settings—are more the rule than the exception. Medication management modalities bear witness to the thesis that the less a therapist considers a patient's psychology, the greater the chance of frame modifications that secretly impair the therapeutic process and outcome. Many pharmacological failures are, at bottom, based on patients' unconsciously mediated adverse reactions to harmful ground rule deviations whose very existence goes unrecognized consciously and yet are replete with negative effects that are deeply felt by both patient and therapist.

SUMMING UP

All in all, then, there is much about the conditions of therapy mandated or implicitly supported by managed care insurers and consciously preferred by managed care psychotherapists that unwittingly promotes departures from the ideal conditions of mental health treatment and a failure to consider the powerful effects of the framework of therapy. There is a strong tendency in managed care therapies, even among dynamically oriented therapists, to allow pragmatism to trump in-depth thinking and consideration of deep unconscious processes and effects. There also is a strong inclination among managed care therapists to focus on their patients' symptoms and gross interpersonal disturbances, on their relatively unrevealing surface communications, and on ways to cognitively modify their emotional difficulties with little thought of their underlying basis. There are few principles of technique with which to guide and validate these healing efforts and a strong inclination to intervene freely in whatever way a therapist believes he or she might be of help to the patient. The practices of psychotherapy and counseling are pretty much matters of laissez-faire these days and there are many indications that much unrecognized harm is being done to both patients and their therapists in this way. Efforts to set matters straight have come mainly from the adaptive approach, a form of psychodynamic therapy to which I now turn.

Chapter Two

The Adaptive Approach

The adaptive approach is based on an empirically grounded, adaptation-oriented listening and formulating process that includes a requisite for the unconscious validation of therapists' interventions and thereby, the formulations on which they are based. The approach has generated a comprehensive understanding of the structure and operations of the human *emotion-processing mind*, the language-based, biological entity that has evolved to adapt to emotionally charged events. Uniquely, the approach draws on archetypal psychobiological principles that have been derived from the science of evolution, which is devoted to the study of both the evolution of biological entities and the nature of their current adaptive resources.

Much like the immune system, which has evolved to enable us to cope with microscopic predators, the emotion-processing mind is a two-system entity that has evolved mainly to cope with trauma-causing macroscopic predators in the form of other humans (and oneself) as well as natural disasters. The emotion-processing mind has a *conscious system* that operates on the basis of conscious perceptions and engages in adaptive efforts of which we are, by and large, directly aware, and a *deep unconscious system* that operates on the basis of unconscious or subliminal perceptions and engages in efforts at adaptation of which we have no direct awareness whatsoever. The perceptions and adaptive operations of this system are encoded in narratives like dreams and stories, which require adaptation-oriented decoding—a process called *trigger decoding*—in order to bring these processes into conscious awareness.

The two systems of the emotion-processing mind operate on the basis of very different resources and defenses, and they do so quite independently of each other. In the main, the conscious system is geared toward denial and defense and its adaptive strategies are therefore compromised and adaptively unreliable. In contrast, the deep unconscious system is relatively non-defensive and open to the most anxiety-provoking meanings of evocative incidents, large and small; its adaptive strategies are incisive and highly effective. Accessing the sound adaptive solutions of this system through trigger decoding is the key to both insightfully resolving emotional symptoms and structuring a sound foundation for a psychotherapy experience—the wisdom of the deep unconscious mind is almost boundless.

All in all, then, consciously orchestrated modes of therapy are likely to be misguided and often deeply harmful. In contrast, therapies structured on the basis of unconsciously validated, trigger-decoded readings of patients' deep unconscious adaptive responses to emotionally charged incidents and their meanings tend to offer a reliable basis for emotional healing. With this in mind, I turn now to the main features of the approach.

THE PILLARS OF THE ADAPTIVE APPROACH

The pillars on which the adaptive approach stands are (Langs 2004, 2006, 2008):

First, the recognition that the emotion-processing mind has important encoding capacities that utilize the mechanisms of displacement, symbolization, and condensation. The adaptive version of this thesis, which is derived from Freud's (1900) theory of dream-formation, differs from the classical psychoanalytic version. The latter proposes that these mechanisms of disguise are applied primarily to forbidden inner wishes and needs. To the contrary, the adaptive position is that the prime targets for disguise are experiences of traumatic external events and their most anxiety-provoking, largely death-related meanings.

Second, the proposition that intellectualizations and narratives are very different modes of expression. The former are single-message communications devoid of disguised meanings, while the latter are double-message communications with both manifest and encoded meanings.

This leads to a third basic proposal to the effect that this communicative distinction points to the existence of two very different operational systems within the emotion-processing mind. The first system is the aforementioned *conscious system* whose adaptive efforts are available to awareness and reflected in the manifest contents of both intellectualizations and narratives like dreams. The second is the *deep unconscious system* whose adaptive efforts are not directly accessible to conscious awareness, but are reflected in the encoded meanings of narrative imagery alone.

The fourth basic thesis is that, as humans, we experience the world and live our lives within two very different realms of experience and in two very different ways—consciously and deep unconsciously. The conscious world of experience is accessed by ascertaining the manifest and implied meanings of intellectualizations and of the surface of narrative material. The deep unconscious world of experience is accessed solely through the already noted process of trigger decoding—ascertaining the disguised meanings of narrative communications in light of the activating triggering events to which the deep unconscious mind is responding adaptively.

These are the foundational, clinically derived concepts on which the adaptive approach is built. The essential features of the approach begin with its reality oriented listening process in which the anxiety-provoking meanings of traumatic events are seen as the central issue in emotional life and its psychotherapy. This insight was derived mainly from the above-mentioned discovery that humans make use of two distinctive modes of communication—*intellectualized* and *narrative*. In essence, intellectualizations are single-message expressions whose manifest contents are fraught with *directly extractable implications that are consciously intended or superficially unconscious, in that while they are not manifest, they are easily detected*. On the other hand, narratives in the form of dreams or stories are double-message communications: One message also is *manifest and consciously intended*, while the other is *encoded, deeply unconscious, and conveyed without an awareness of its contents*. These heavily disguised latter meanings are reflections of unconscious adaptive responses to anxiety-provoking, death-related, traumatic triggering events whose implications and impact are too anxiety-provoking to register in conscious awareness. In some situations, an entire traumatic incident is quickly erased from awareness and becomes irretrievable to conscious recall. In other cases, the most anxiety-provoking meanings of consciously experienced events do not register in awareness and therefore are unavailable to conscious awareness. These meanings are unconsciously registered and they are revealed solely through encoded narrative imagery, most often in the form of dreams and guided narrative associations to their elements. It is here that trigger decoding comes into play—the unmasking of the disguised meanings of a narrative image in light of the traumatic triggering event that has evoked it.

For patients in psychotherapy, severe traumas outside of treatment may at times be the source of deep unconscious experiences and encoded narrative images, but in most instances the disturbing triggers that are processed by patients' deep unconscious systems involve the implications and meanings of their therapists' interventions. In this regard, it has been found that many seemingly innocent interventions, including all manner of departures from the ideal framework of treatment, that are thought to be innocuous and thus accepted consciously by patients—and their therapists—are experienced deep unconsciously as evocative of some form of death anxiety and harmful to the patient (and therapist) as well. Even frame-securing interventions—efforts to institute the ideal archetypal frame—while basically healing, usually evoke forms of death anxiety, largely existential in nature. This finding accounts in part for the conscious preference in both therapists and patients for modified frames that preclude the experience of this dreaded form of angst.

A NEW MODEL OF THE MIND

A major feature of the adaptive approach is its revised model of the mind as a language-based *emotion-processing mental module* that has evolved to adapt to emotionally charged events that are consciously or unconsciously experienced as traumatic and death-related (Langs, 2004, 2006). As noted, the module is comprised of two relatively independent operating systems: A *conscious system* whose adaptive processing efforts register or are able to register in awareness and a *deep unconscious system* whose adaptive efforts have no direct access to awareness but are conveyed solely through the encoded meanings of narrative expressions.

Both systems operate cognitively on the basis of perceptions—conscious or subliminal/unconscious—of the meanings and implications of triggering events. However, the conscious system is geared toward defense and the denial of death and thus fails to perceive many emotionally threatening incidents and their meanings. The resultant loss of information and knowledge severely compromises the system's adaptive resources and efforts; indeed, emotion-related conscious intelligence is severely impaired.

To make matters worse, the conscious system's malfunctioning is aggravated because it also is under the influence of deep unconscious guilt which unwittingly biases conscious thinking and behaviors toward choices that are unwittingly self-punitive and self-defeating. The system's frame-related preferences, which lean strongly toward departures from the ideal archetypal frame, are a major case in point as seen in the finding that even as these choices are embraced consciously, they are validly perceived unconsciously as distinctly self-harmful.

In contrast to the conscious mind, the deep unconscious system operates on the basis of an openness of perception that has provided it with an enormously rich, effective adaptive wisdom that enables it to consistently make wise, archetypal adaptive choices that are, as noted, encoded in narrative responses to triggering events. The system is highly sensitive to the consciously obliterated, death-related, and other anxiety-provoking meanings of disruptive events and thus with full vision arrives at appropriate adaptive choices, such as those pertaining to securing the ground rules of treatment. It is a system whose adaptive preferences are optimally enhancing for oneself and fully respectful of the needs and feelings of others.

Both systems of the mind have subsystems of morality and ethics. Conscious morality is highly individualized and easily compromised, as seen in the rampant corruption that exists in the world today and in the not infrequent overtly dishonest arrangements that managed care therapists have made. There are many unconscious sources of this conscious system tendency to turn to corrupt frame violations; most of them involve the death anxiety evoked by secured frames and the unconscious belief that death is defeated through frame violations (see below). In contrast, deep unconscious morality is based on an archetypal, universal moral code that is pristine and uncompromising—and consistently advocated. The system enforces this ideal code of ethics and behavior by unconsciously orchestrating punishments for violations of its principles and rewards for adherence to its tenets.

The conscious mind's responses to emotionally charged incidents are highly individualized and thus arriving at a conscious consensus about the best way to deal with an emotionally charged issue, be it a conscious conflict or question regarding a ground rule of therapy, is all but impossible. Deep unconscious decisions are a very different matter because the system's viewpoint, understanding, and choices are archetypal—that is, universally shared—and thus single-minded. In psychotherapy, trigger decoding patients' narratives themes when a frame issue arises or when a ground is invoked or modified always points to securing the optimal frame under the prevailing conditions. There is, then, no sound reason to make frame-related decisions based on conscious thinking when trigger decoding will reveal the ideal archetypal frame. This is especially necessary when it comes to the ground rules and boundaries of managed care therapies largely because it requires the participants to therapy to work under conditions that are compromised framewise, a situation that creates pressures for further frame modifications that can best be curtailed through accessing deep unconscious choices through trigger decoding.

THE ROLE OF DEATH AND DEATH ANXIETY

In turning to the traumas and emotion-related threats posed by reality, it becomes clear that death and the anxieties it evokes in us as humans is by far the greatest source of danger we experience in both our lives and the psychotherapy of its emotional ills. Because the conscious mind has evolved largely to deny death and the death-related meanings of many traumas, including many that are psychological and frame-related, and because most of the death-related meanings of everyday events are experienced deep unconsciously, we tend to have little or no appreciation of the pervasiveness of our concerns about death and the amount of death anxiety we experience each day of our lives. While death and death-related anxieties may at times be experienced consciously, *unconscious death anxiety* is much like the invisible background radiation that has filled the universe after its creation through the big bang—it is everywhere at all times. It is left to the deep unconscious mind to detect the presence of most of the death-related meanings and anxieties that are evoked by disturbing triggering events. It is the therapist's task to trigger decode their patients' dreams and stories to discover the presence of these issues—and with that, the adaptive solutions that are being recommended by their highly sensitive deep unconscious minds.

There are three forms of death anxiety (Langs 1997, 2006, 2008). Each form is, in most instances, perceived and experienced unconsciously and each tends to have major, unconsciously mediated consequences. The three forms are:

Predatory death anxiety—the fear of psychological and/or physical harm from natural disasters or at the hands of other living beings, especially other humans. The basic response to this form of death anxiety is a mobilization of resources generated to defend against the threat at hand. In respect to the rules, frames, and boundaries of psychotherapy, all departures from the archetypal frame are experienced deep unconsciously as damaging and thus as evocative of this form of death anxiety.

Therapists tend to invoke frame modifications based on their deep unconscious need to deny their vulnerability to death and to empower themselves on the basis of the unconscious belief that those who harm others are immune to being harmed themselves. As for their part, patients unwittingly accept their therapists' predatory frame violations because of their deep unconscious guilt and need for punishment and because they prefer to deal with predatory death anxiety rather than the existential form which would be evoked in a secured frame. The unconscious thinking behind this preference is that they can combat and possibly defeat predators, but there is no effective way of defeating the inevitability of personal death.

Predator death anxiety—the fear of retribution by death for harm caused to others. This type of death anxiety is evoked by deep unconscious guilt and leads to needs for punishment. As a result, the deep unconscious mind silently orchestrates self-defeating decisions and behaviors in order to satisfy this need. This form of death anxiety is responsible for many departures from the archetypically ideal frame in that therapists often modify one or more ground rules in guilt-ridden unconscious, predatory efforts to have their patients punish them in some manner for the harm that they have caused others. On their side, patients tend to accept or ask for these frame deviations largely because of their own unconscious need to be harmed and punished for the damage they have done to others.

Existential death anxiety—the fear connected with the inevitability of personal death and the death of those with whom a person has a special relationship. The basic response to this form of death anxiety is conscious denial and obliteration, mechanisms that come in a myriad of guises, behavioral and psychological. Most of the existential death anxieties to which humans are subjected are triggered by traumas, psychological and physical, whose significant meanings and implications tend to not register in conscious awareness. These death-related meanings are instead experienced and adaptively processed deep unconsciously.

This form of death anxiety is a major unconsciously mediated cause of unnecessary frame modifications. This is the case because secured frames—that is, therapies in which all of the archetypal ground rules have been established and prevail—arouse intense entrapment and thus existential death anxieties in both parties to treatment. In consequence, both therapists and their patients are consciously inclined toward frame modifications as a way of dissipating their existential fears. There is an essentially delusional unconscious belief in all humans that individuals who can defy an archetypal ground rule can defy the basic existential, biologically determined ground rule that life is followed by death. Humans have given up their lives trying in vain to prove that this is the case.

There is, then, a set of relatively fixed connections between death anxiety and the deep unconscious experience of ground-rule-related conditions and interventions. *Secured frames*, in which all of the fundamental, archetypal, deep unconsciously sought and validated ground rules are in place, and *secured frame moments*, in which a modified ground rule is rectified for one or more sessions, offer optimally healing and inherently supportive conditions for a therapeutic experience, but they also evoke entrapping, existential death anxieties. This is a universal phenomenon experienced deep unconsciously by both patients and therapists. And this type of anxiety, which is modeled on the realization that we are born into a closed space from which death is the only exit, has an enormous, albeit unconscious, influence on conscious thinking and the ground rule choices made by both patients and therapists in structuring and sustaining a psychotherapy experience.

Denial of the inevitability of death and relief from its attendant anxieties are, then, effected though departures from the archetypal frame. Because the conscious mind is so denial-prone, managed care frames whose ground rules have been modified beyond the deviations mandated by insurers are more the rule than the exception. These frame breaks offer a temporary sense of relief but they also are harmful to all concerned. They tend to promote a turn to additional damaging frame violations within the therapy and in the everyday lives of both parties to treatment. Still, the intensity of secured-frame, existential death anxieties is so great that quite unwittingly, the conscious minds of both patients and therapists tend to prefer deviant rather than secured frame conditions. Temporary immediate relief is gained at the cost of losing the curative qualities of the secured frame.

SOME BASIC PERSPECTIVES

One of the most startling conclusions to be drawn from adaptive studies of the emotion-processing mind is that the conscious mind is, by evolved design, quite incapable of defining and validating the ideal conditions under which managed care psychotherapy—or any other type of emotion-related healing—should be carried out. With only rare exceptions, conscious minds tend to seek compromised forms of emotional relief, much of it paradoxically through damaging rather than healing frames. In addition, the conscious mind has not garnered the necessary frame-related knowledge to craft the ideal conditions for treatment. Indeed, this lack of wisdom applies to the most sophisticated psychoanalytically oriented therapists because of their manifestly centered listening processes. The only way to arrive at the ideal, archetypal frame is to engage in trigger decoding in order to access the thinking and adaptive preferences of the deep unconscious mind. Short of that, anything goes and the conscious choices made by therapists and patients alike almost always are more damaging than enabling for both of them.

There are several features of the conscious system that renders it all but incapable of identifying and securing the ideal frame. The system suffers gravely from existential death anxiety and unwittingly resorts to an endless array of obliterating, self-deceptive defensive mechanisms in order to deny the inevitability of personal death—frame modifications chief among them. The conscious mind also is unable to appreciate the encoded attributes of narrative communications and it is naturally disinclined to engage in trigger decoding, the process that would yield the frame-related insights that the conscious mind is unable to generate on its own. Relevant too is the enormous influence that predator death anxiety and deep unconscious guilt exerts on the conscious mind. There is a powerful deep unconscious need in patients and therapists to find ways to punish themselves for harm they have done to others. This unconsciously mediated need skews their frame-related decisions toward harmful frame modifications that are self-punitive and invite punishment from the other party to therapy. Self-punitive needs are seldom satisfied in this way—the deep unconscious system of morality and ethics demands many acts of unconsciously wrought repentance and redemption before it relents in its punitive activities. The result tends to be a vicious circle in which deep unconscious guilt provokes the turn to unnecessary, bilaterally damaging frame violations which then cause fresh deep unconscious guilt and further need for punitive frame modifications in both parties to the therapy. In most situations, however, the prime mover is the therapist who thereby suffers from predator death anxiety, while the willing victim is the patient who experiences considerable predatory death anxiety as a result.

A system of the mind that is dominated by needs of this kind is too dysfunctional to choose the best possible available conditions for a psychotherapy experience. Lacking archetypes and a reliable means of validating frame-related interventions, maladaptive conscious preferences prevail—much of them under the influence of an individual's history of death-related traumas. This realization is an extension of the broader adaptive insight that the conscious mind is so dysfunctionally constructed that it is incapable of defining the features of the ideal form of psychotherapy. This means that patients are unable consciously to choose the best possible therapist for their psychotherapy experience—only the deep unconscious system alone knows how to do this.

In order to define the ideal frame of managed care therapy, then, we must, as I have been emphasizing, turn to the second system of the emotion-processing mind, the deep unconscious system. This system operates without conscious awareness largely because it experiences the most morbid and anxiety-provoking aspects of human behaviors and triggering events, aspects that are intolerable to conscious awareness. The deep unconscious system is extremely sensitive to the consciously obliterated death-related meanings of triggering events and also is highly principled morally; it possesses and operates on the basis of the wisdom and morality needed to define and seek the archetypically healing, ideal framework for a therapy experience. Because the system is able to perceive death-related threats it can develop the adaptive strategies that are needed to cope effectively with the relevant anxieties. But this adaptive wisdom does not enter awareness directly because it is based on and linked to our most dreaded traumas, hurts, and moments of utter helplessness. The adaptive mastery of death and a tolerance of secured frames, which come naturally to the deep unconscious mind, requires intense, repetitive efforts at trigger decoding in order to become part of the repertoire of the conscious mind.

A CLINICAL ILLUSTRATION

I shall close this chapter with a brief vignette from a managed care psychotherapy experience presented to me by Dr. Tyler, a woman psychologist whose work I was supervising. Her patient, a man I shall call Mr. Thomas, began a session in the second year of his therapy with a dream in which he's in Iraq. The details were vague but he immediately thought of a newspaper story he had read on the day of the dream in which a woman terrorist blew herself up at a check point, killing herself, several civilians, and the two American soldiers who were supposed to be protecting them. It turned out that a warning of the danger of a terrorist attack had been sent to the soldiers but the message had been ignored.

There were other associations to the violence in Iraq and indications that the patient had experienced a high level of anxiety during the past week, but none of the additional incidents he mentioned enabled either him or the therapist to identify the trigger—most likely a recent intervention made by Dr. Tyler—that had evoked this morbid dream. She announced that the session was at an end and Mr. Thomas stood up and took out a letter from the insurance company, waved it in the air, and mentioned that he hadn't had time to look into the problem—adding that he would do so later that week. With that, the patient left the office.

The letter in question was a second notice to the patient that the therapist had failed to obtain authorization for the sessions held the previous month. Until Mr. Thomas took out the letter, Dr. Tyler, who had received both notices, had completely blotted out her conscious awareness of both letters. She had, then, not as yet contacted the insurance company to find out how to set the matter straight.

Consciously, the patient had treated this matter as having little significance and despite the threat it posed to the continuation of his treatment, he hadn't brought up either notice in any of his sessions. For her part, the therapist had totally forgotten that she needed to send in a request for authorization for additional sessions and she also blocked out the two letters despite her realization when she read them that, left unresolved, this matter could destroy the therapy.

The dream and especially the patient's associations to the dream include encoded bridging themes that link the narrative images to these triggering events—Dr. Tyler's lapse, which included her failure to send in the necessary form, her not responding to the first notice, and not bringing up the second notice in the session just described. The patient's deep unconscious experience of the implications of these interventional lapses are disguised in the allusions to someone destroying herself and others and in the supposedly protective soldiers ignoring a warning message that spoke of a potentially fatal attack.

During the session, these encoded themes, which point to triggers to which the patient had not alluded to manifestly, had not, as they should have, modified the therapist's obliterating defenses. As a result, she was unable to work interpretively with this material with an eye toward her securing the frame and providing deep insight for the patient. By and large therapists need to be aware of the triggers for patients' narrative themes in order to properly trigger decode and act on the basis of their disguised meanings.

That night, Dr. Tyler decided to engage in private self-processing—the adaptive form of self-analysis (Langs 1993, 2006). She wanted to understand the unconscious reasons she had failed to send the form to the insurance company; this is a so-called indicator of an emotional problem whose deep unconscious sources in triggering events and their deep unconscious meanings needed to be ascertained. She first went directly to her conscious feelings and recognized that Mr. Thomas was a very difficult patient whom she might well have been trying unconsciously to terminate. But realizing that this was a mundane, unempowered, intellectualized, conscious system explanation of little consequence, she recalled the dream fragment she had had the previous night, soon after her lapse had been brought to her attention.

In the dream an elderly man was lying in a gutter, face-down with a knife in his side. The main associations were to her father who had collapsed on the street two months earlier. It turned out that he had suffered a second heart attack and that she was worried that he would not survive this episode. She was plagued with guilt over being a rebellious daughter and over the fact that his first heart attack occurred soon after she had quarreled with him. In recent months the tension between them had increased over her interest in a man who was of a religion different from hers.

Dr. Tyler could now see that her failure to send in the form was a reaction to these death-related traumas. They had affected her work by unconsciously motivating an acting out on her part that created a situation in which the life of Mr. Thomas' therapy (and by implication of both the patient and herself) was at stake. She also had put herself in the position of having to turn to extraordinary measures to resuscitate the patient and his treatment and ensure their survival. In addition, her lapse was an unconsciously driven attempt to punish herself for the harm she had caused her father by provoking and losing the patient—events that would cause her much suffering.

Having recognized the triggers that had unconsciously evoked her lapses and the triggers for her patient's dream of, and associations to Iraq, Dr. Tyler was now able to proceed to contact the insurance company and set in motion the necessary steps to obtaining approval for continuing the therapy. She also was able in the following session to trigger decode and interpret a fresh dream from the patient in which a woman from work who despises him tries to blow up Mr. Thomas' house.

Therapists' insights into and resolution of their own sources of secured-frame death anxieties are a requisite for their working insightfully and toward securing modified frames when their patients are suffering from very similar issues. For therapists, then, healing themselves is the first step on the road to deeply healing their patients.

The deep unconscious mind knows full well that frame-related lapses always are a consequence of an active, contemporary death-related triggering event that has taken place inside or outside of therapy. For patients, the relevant trauma most often is perpetrated by their therapists, while for therapists, the trauma more often takes place in their everyday lives. Along different lines, we see that blatant frame violations such as this therapist's repeated lapses are typically experienced deep unconsciously and with great validity in the most gruesome ways possible. This is characteristic of the wisdom of the deep unconscious mind—it is grimly conveyed, but entirely in the service of therapeutic healing. With this in mind, I turn now the archetypal ground rules of psychotherapy as a yardstick against which I shall then take the measure of the managed care frame.

Chapter Three

The Archetypal Ground Rules of Psychotherapy

Studies of the evolution of the emotion-processing mind and its current mode of adaptation have led to the discovery that, as humans, we naturally wish to live our lives, interact emotionally with others, and do our psychotherapy within a particular kind of well-defined, integrated framework. Much as lungs do best in an environment rich with oxygen, the emotion-processing mind—and we ourselves—do best emotionally under a specific set of environmental conditions.

There are, however, a series of fateful differences between lungs and emotion-processing minds. Driven by a biological need for survival, we unhesitatingly, and without inner restraint, relentlessly seek the ideal conditions for breathing. But when it comes to the ideal conditions for emotionally meaningful interactions and the process of emotional healing, we are strikingly disinclined to consciously seek the much-needed optimal framework. Instead, we are of divided minds: Universally and by evolved design, we are, in general, consciously reluctant to operate under secured-frame conditions, yet all the while, we wish deep unconsciously to do so (Langs 1998, 2004, 2006, 2008). But unless we engage in trigger decoding encoded messages, we not only are unaware of this unconscious preference, we also do not behave accordingly. The human mind is not well designed for emotion-related adaptations.

Geared for sustaining psychological defenses against death anxiety in particular, both patients and therapists consciously tend to ignore or disregard frame conditions and accept or prefer modified rather than ideally secured frames—in both psychotherapy and their everyday lives. Thoughtlessly, they are consciously inclined to seek poor or harmful—costly, yet defensively protective—frame-related conditions even as they generate mostly unrecognized encoded narratives that speak for the ideal conditions that they manifestly disregard and avoid. By and large, conscious preferences, which are unconsciously affected by the need to deny death and by the search for ways to harm and punish oneself for having harmed others, tend to hold sway. This is the case because our deep unconscious preferences are unknown to awareness and therefore do not affect our conscious choices. These maladaptive conscious preferences make doing and receiving managed care psychotherapy, which is carried out within a mandated deviant frame, a most risky undertaking in which the possibilities of frame-related harm looms quite large.

THE BASIC FRAMES

Secured Frames

The archetypal conditions for psychotherapy define what is known as *the secured frame. This frame is defined as the set of ground rules and boundaries that are consistently and essentially without exception validated deep unconsciously through patients' encoded responses to frame-related triggering events*—that is, to moments when a therapist establishes, sustains, or modifies one or more of the ground rules and boundaries of a psychotherapy experience. Broadly stated, affirmative disguised themes support a therapist's frame-related interventions, while harmful themes refute these efforts. The archetypal frame is, then, that set of ground rules that are universally affirmed through the patient's encoded imagery when a frame issue is activated.

The concept of psychological universals or archetypes was championed by Jung (1968). He did not, however, identify and explore the archetypes related to rules, frames, and boundaries or those that pertain to experiencing and coping with death and death anxiety. Because today's therapists are conscious-system therapists whose observations are confined to manifest contents and their implications, they tend to think of the human mind and therapeutic interactions in terms that stress individuality and the differences that exist from one person and therapeutic dyad to the next. This individuality is characteristic of the conscious mind and conscious thinking. Thus, while there is an evolved, universal design of the conscious system, its adaptive operations are not based on archetypes but are highly individualized. They vary greatly from one person to the next, much of it based on factors such as biological givens, various current conditions, psychological preferences, needs for defense and denial, and a person's trauma-related history. These individual preferences characterize conscious system thinking and make it impossible to consciously define the ideal, secured frame for managed care and other forms of psychotherapy. As noted, this important goal can be achieved solely through trigger decoding and accessing deep unconscious archetype-based needs and preferences.

Basically, then, a *secured-frame psychotherapy experience* is one in which all of the archetypal ground rules are put into place and sustained with the support of a patient's encoded images as derived from his or her deep unconscious responses to frame-related triggering events. In addition, when working within a modified frame, a deviant ground rule may be rectified, often at the behest of a patient's encoded directives. This type of intervention creates a lasting or temporary *secured-frame moment or interlude*, one that evokes both the salutary experiences connected with the invocation of the ideal frame as well *the deep unconscious secured-frame death anxieties* that always accompany these positive effects.

While a managed care psychotherapy experience cannot by definition take place within an ideal secured frame, it can transpire in a setting where the frame modifications are kept to an absolute minimum. Clinical experience indicates that such frames tend to hold patients well and are more healing than damaging, and that the contracted modifications of the managed care ground rules tend in these cases to recede into the background. This holds true unless something happens to reactivate the impact of a mandated deviant ground rule. An example of this phenomenon is seen when a therapist is required to send a treatment report to the insurance company in order to obtain authorization for further sessions. This request will re-arouse a patient's issues pertaining to the absence of total privacy and confidentiality for the therapy and the effects of these departures from the ideal frame will then need to be reworked and resolved to the greatest extent feasible under the prevailing conditions.

Modified Frames

Treatment experiences that are conducted under conditions that depart in one or more ways from the unconsciously validated archetypal framework of treatment are deviant-frame or frame-modified psychotherapies. By definition and mandate, managed care psychotherapy is carried out under this second type of frame condition. We therefore need to know as much as possible about the effects of these conditions and how to limit and resolve those consequences that are most detrimental to both managed care patients and their therapists—and the insurers who sponsor and oversee their therapeutic work.

Without exception, managed care patients come to a psychotherapy or medication consultation consciously prepared to accept frame-modified conditions for their treatment experience. In addition, because of strong unconscious influences, most patients expect that their managed care therapists will invoke a wide range of additional departures from the archetypal frame—patients tend to consciously accept or seek as many frame modifications as they can tolerate, rationalize, or ignore. We need to be mindful, however, that these conscious preferences hold sway in the face of strong but encoded objections from their deep unconscious minds.

The situation is even more perfidious than this preference suggests because of the problems that tend to arise when a ground rule that can be secured comes up as an issue in managed care psychotherapy. At such times the patient's encoded imagery, if allowed expression, always confirms the need to change and optimize the ground rule in question. But given the current manifest-content approaches to psychotherapy, in most instances this deep unconscious affirmation goes unrecognized, uninterpreted, and unutilized. But even if the trigger decoded interpretation is made, at the very moment when the therapist proposes to secure the ground rule in question as per the patient's encoded imagery, many managed care patients will raise conscious objections to this decision and turn against the therapist and therapy. Not infrequently, this secured-frame moment creates unbearable unconscious existential death anxieties in the patient, who will then, without being consciously aware of his or her unconscious reasons, terminate their therapy. The dread of the secured frame is especially problematic with managed care patients because the inherently deviant managed care frame seems to assure them that they are not likely to experience the dreaded—but therapeutically workable and resolvable—existential death anxieties that a secured ground rule generates.

A common example of this kind of reaction arises when, based on a patient's encoded directives, a therapist changes the ground rule of responsibility for sessions from a flexible rule that allows, with advance notice, non-payment for some missed sessions to one in which the patient is responsible for the fee for all missed sessions. This archetypal ground rule provides patients with essential healing experiences related to commitment, responsibility, necessary restraint, and therapeutic holding in lieu of the therapist abandoning and demeaning the patient by permitting him or her to freely miss sessions. It also assures the therapist who has reserved the time of the patient's sessions that he or she will be paid for this time and not lose income when the patient misses the hour.

Goaded unconsciously by their existential death anxieties, however, many patients object to this secured ground rule. Some of them refuse to accept it as a condition for treatment, acting as if they have no consistent responsibility to the therapist or therapy for the fee for their sessions and that the therapist rather than they should suffer the financial loss involved in a missed hour for which insurers do not pay. Their abuse of the therapist is entirely overlooked by their conscious mind, but they nonetheless experience deep unconscious guilt for harming the therapist—guilt which will unconsciously motivate patients to punitively harm themselves in some way—acts and choices that go unrecognized for what they are because their sources operate outside of awareness. On the other hand, it is not uncommon for patients who agree to this frame-securing intervention to unconsciously experience existential entrapment anxieties that prompt them to uninsightfully quit therapy soon after doing so (see chapter six).

In like fashion, managed care patients who can afford to move to private therapy and who encode the advisability of such a change also show enormous resistances to doing so. Quite often, they find a conscious excuse or rationalization as a basis for terminating their therapy instead of seeing the therapist privately. All in all, the first secured-frame moment in the course of a managed care treatment experience—should any occur—is a crisis moment for the therapy and regardless of whether it is explored or ignored by the therapist, patients often precipitously take flight from the therapy.

These trends bear witness to the pervasive dread in humans of the existential death anxieties evoked by secured frames and secured-frame moments. Managed care patients have a strong, albeit unconscious, investment in doing psychotherapy under deviant-frame conditions so as to cover over and defend against, rather than process and adapt to, the existential death anxieties that always play a role in emotional maladaptations. It is well to appreciate then that without a secured-frame moment, these anxieties and the death-related traumas on which they are based do not become available for exploration and resolution. As a result, they continue to be a major unconscious cause of symptoms in patients who unwittingly deal with these issues in maladaptive, self-harmful, frame-modifying fashion. In managed care therapy, secured-frame moments create special opportunities for insightful healing even as they pose an enormous threat to the continuation of treatment.

THE ARCHETYPAL COMPONENTS OF THE SECURED FRAME

Thirty years of studying both secured and modified psychotherapy frames under a variety of conditions including managed care enables me to define the presently known components of the archetypal, deep unconsciously sought, optimally healing, inherently supportive framework for a psychotherapy experience (Langs 2004, 2006). I shall do so using as my basic standard the one-to-one, private psychotherapy situation. The following are the main ground rules and setting components of the ideal, secured frame:

1. *An uncontaminated referral to the therapist of a individual who does not know the therapist personally nor has had prior social or any other kind of contact with him or her. In addition, the referral is professional in nature in that it has been made by a physician, mental health professional, or someone with similar qualifications. Patient-referrals are thereby precluded.*

The secured frame calls for an impersonal, professional referral as a way of providing the interpersonal boundaries and relative anonymity of the therapist that are vital to a soundly holding frame. This ground rule restricts the therapist from seeing in consultation or accepting for therapy any person who has personal knowledge of his or her private life or who has had a prior social or professional contact with him or her. Managed care referrals can and often do meet this requirement, largely because patients tend to make their initial contact with a therapist based on a list of providers that does not include personal information about the therapist.

2. *A professional setting with a soundproofed office and a waiting room that is used exclusively by the therapist. The décor is neutral, with no family memorabilia or other personal items.*

This type of office setting can readily be created and used by managed care psychotherapists. There is, however, an economically rationalized but unconsciously driven, defensive tendency related to personal death-related traumas and anxieties that motivate many therapists to make use of frame-modifying shared office spaces with shared waiting rooms or to establish offices on the grounds of their homes or apartments. These office settings are frame-deviant.

3. *A set time, length, and frequency of sessions—aspects of the so-called fixed or stable frame.*

These elements of the ideal frame can and should be adopted by managed care psychotherapists as a way of providing an important measure of regularity to the foundation for the patient's psychotherapy experience.

4. *A single, set fee commensurate with a therapist's expertise, one that is paid for by the patient alone.*

This is one of the ideal ground rules and aspect of the fixed frame that is inherently compromised in managed care situations by the provision that the insurer pay the therapist part or all of the fee for services. In addition, because managed care fees tend to be below therapists' usual and customary private fees, these payments seldom are in keeping with the level of a therapist's expertise.

5. *Full responsibility for both parties to be present for all scheduled sessions.*

Some managed care insurers modify this ground rule by mandating that therapists allow patients to cancel sessions with 24- or 48-hour advance notice. Neither the patient nor the insurer bear any responsibility for the therapist's fee for these missed hours—insurers do not pay for services that are not rendered. On the other hand, the therapist's responsibility to attend regularly scheduled session can and should be sustained in managed care psychotherapy.

6. *The therapist's prerogative and responsibility to take occasional extended vacations that are announced well in advance.*

This ground rule can and should be followed by managed care psychotherapists without modification. Therapists' judicious, planned absences from therapy are interruptions of the therapeutic process, but they are frame securing in that a therapist who does not take time off each year is unduly entrapping the patient and thus, being frame-deviant in a most unusual manner.

7. *Total privacy, with no contact or involvement with outside (third) parties by the therapist or patient.*

This is one of the more crucial archetypal ground rules of psychotherapy but it cannot be enforced in managed care settings, which, by definition, involve the release of information by providers to insurers. These revelations range from transmitting a patient's diagnosis and dates of service, which is the very minimum, to being mandated to provide a detailed progress report regarding the transactions and status of the treatment. Under some circumstances, insurers ask managed care therapists to provide them with copies of their process notes. Along different lines, requests also may be made by both patients and insurers to release information to other third parties such as a patient's employer, employment assistance providers, disability providers, and other professionals who are treating a particular patient. To safeguard the patient and the therapy to the greatest extent feasible, these deviations should, however, be kept to an absolute minimum.

8. *Total confidentiality, with no note-taking or recording of the transactions of the sessions by either party to treatment, and no release of information of any kind.*

This too is a ground rule that cannot be adhered to in managed care settings. Because privacy and confidentiality tend to go hand in hand, the comments made above regarding privacy tend to apply to confidentiality as well. In addition, federal and state statutes and most managed care insurers have regulations that mandate therapist's note-taking and record-keeping for a managed care psychotherapy experience. In these situations, therapists must adhere to these requirements even though they violate the ideal rules for privacy and confidentiality; only a minimal amount of information should be recorded.

9. *The relative anonymity of the therapist, who restrains from making deliberate (as distinct from inescapable) self-revelations and from offering advice, personal opinions, directives, extraneous remarks, and the like.*

This ground rule, which can be invoked in a managed care psychotherapy, involves the *relative* anonymity of the therapist because therapists are inescapably self-revealing through how they decorate their offices, dress, intervene, and much more. These inevitable self-revelations are not frame modifying, while unnecessary self-revelations and opinions do indeed compromise the ideal frame. Patients also may violate this ground rule by seeking a therapist with whom they have had prior contact or knowledge, or by "Googling" the therapist, checking for information about him or her on-line in the frame-deviant hope of discovering a great deal about the therapist's professional career and, at times, personal life. The powerful unconscious effects of this type of frame violation is attested to by the frequency with which patients knowingly or inadvertently conceal this frame-modifying activity from their therapists and resist exploring its ramifications when their encoded themes point to its having taken place.

10. *The fundamental rule of "free association" (the advice to patients to say whatever comes to mind), supplemented by the rule of "guided associations" (the advice to patients to associate to the elements of their dreams by recalling and recounting—that is, narrating—the incidents from their outside lives that they conjure up).*

These two ground rules, which can be invoked in managed care situations, explicitly facilitate the need for patients to generate the narrative material required for the insightful cure of their emotional maladaptations based on trigger decoding the deep unconscious meanings of these communications. The rule of free association was established by Freud and is used by many dynamically oriented therapists, while the rule of guided associations is invoked by adaptive therapists as a means of fostering the communication of encoded narratives. Even though these rules are not invoked by many therapists and counselors, they nevertheless are deep unconsciously sought, archetypal ideals.

11. *The therapist's use of neutral interventions.*

This is another ground rule that can be adhered to by therapists working under managed care conditions. Neutrality is a theory-driven concept that is defined differently by the various schools of psychotherapy. Nevertheless, the rule implies in principle that, in intervening, a therapist will make exclusive use of the meanings and implications of a patient's material in a given session and not introduce his or her own unneeded and uncalled-for personal biases or offer comments that are not based on the patient's material. Beyond that requisite, it has been found clinically that only sound trigger decoded interpretations and frame-securing interventions obtain *deep unconscious, encoded validation* and thus, that this type of intervention alone is archetypal in nature and universally confirmed.

12. *The absence of physical contact between the two parties to therapy.*

This ground rule also is applicable to—and necessary in—managed care therapies. Its violation in hands-on therapies, while part of that particular treatment regime nonetheless has extensive deep unconsciously mediated, detrimental effects on the patients and therapists who are party to these physical contacts.

13. *Confinement of the contact between the patient and therapist to the time and place of the scheduled sessions.*

This is another ground rule that can be applied in managed care therapy situations. It speaks for the avoidance of outside contact between patient and therapist and precludes their meeting before, during, or after the termination of treatment.

14. *A group of less well defined, implicit ground rules, such as the therapist's primary dedication to the therapeutic needs of the patient and the patient's agreement to listen to and give serious consideration to his or her therapist's interventions.*

Modifications of these less well defined ground rules are not uncommon in the managed care treatment situation. This arises mainly because of the mandated frame modifications of this treatment modality, which dilute the commitment each party to therapy makes to the other party.

SUMMING UP

Summing up, it is quite evident that managed care treatment takes place under less than ideal conditions. The extent to which the mandated frame modifications cause unconsciously mediated harm to both patients and therapists is an open question. Empirically, it has been found that much depends on a therapist's sensitivity to frame issues and the extent to which he or she listens to and interprets patients' encoded material related to the ground rules of treatment and on that basis, secures those archetypal ground rules that can be maintained for the therapy. Indeed, the more secured the frame, the less damage and the more healing the managed care frame provides for both parties to treatment.

In managed care therapies that have been conducted by adaptive psychotherapists, patients' deep unconscious concerns with the deviant conditions of the therapy often fade into the background and tend to cause damage only when a modified rule is used in a destructive manner by either participant to the therapy. By and large, whenever a therapist holds much of the frame steady and secured, and there is no active issue related to the inescapable modified ground rules, the therapeutic work will center around the recovery, often by means of encoded images rather than direct recall, of the patient's most pathogenic death-related traumas as they are activated by the therapist's interventions and the ongoing conditions of treatment—and more rarely, by gross traumas outside of the therapy. This means that in addition to being a guide to the archetypal frame, the encoded messages from the deep unconscious system are the most common means through which patients reveal their core traumas and conflicts, however much disguised; but in addition, they also guide therapists as to how psychotherapy is best conducted—frame-wise and interpretively. While no system in nature is perfect or without its dysfunctions, the deep unconscious system comes close this ideal. With this in mind, I turn now to a closer look at secured and modified psychotherapy frames.

Chapter Four

Secured and Modified Frames

There is much in human life that involves trade-offs. Quite often we are called on to make choices for which a cost in emotional pain or suffering is inevitable no matter which way we go. Many frame-related decisions made by psychotherapists and their patients, be it securing or modifying a ground rule, have both advantages and disadvantages. The down side may be either unnecessarily or inevitably harmful, but in either case it also may in time be turned to therapeutic advantage. As the saying goes, the parties to managed care psychotherapy often find themselves between a rock and a hard place. For both patient and therapist, adhering to or securing a ground rule will be healing deep unconsciously, yet it often is the cause of unconscious anxieties that activate severe conscious resistances. On the other hand, opting for a modified ground rule is consistently harmful deep unconsciously, yet often temporarily anxiety-relieving and welcomed consciously by both patients and therapists. The handling of the framework of psychotherapy, and managed care therapy in particular, is a constant source of disturbing dilemmas and difficult decisions.

THE EFFECTS OF SECURED FRAMES

Turning first to deep unconsciously validated secured frames, they are fundamentally healing because they offer patients and their therapists safety, security, inherent support, a sense of mutual trust, the avoidance of unnecessary, self-harmful deep unconscious guilt, and a favorable context that reinforces a therapist's sound verbal and other constructive interventions. At the same time, however, the ideal ground rules are limiting and restrictive.

These inescapable, frustrating, and entrapping qualities arouse terrifying deep unconscious existential death anxieties in both patients and therapists because entrapment anxieties are basic to human life and its inevitable end in death. Indeed, *the fundamental, existential rule of life* states that we are born into a circumscribed space from which we, as humans, can exit only through our personal demise.

Despite the deep unconscious anxieties that are evoked by secured-frame conditions, this is the only frame that offers patients the unique therapeutic opportunity to experience, express, and gain insight into the very same existential death anxieties that are, without exception, one of the root causes of their emotional pain and suffering. Even so, dealing with encoded expressions of these anxieties—and most of the more significant experiences of death anxiety, current and past, are experienced unconsciously rather than consciously—meets with many resistances in patients and counter-resistances in their therapists. Thus, even though the healing qualities of secured frames are validated by patients' deep unconscious minds and are reflected in the alleviation of patients' symptoms (for some patients, securing the archetypal frame does all of the healing), and even though they begin to cope better emotionally, conscious inclinations in patients to resist or flee the secured frame psychotherapy are not uncommon after a frame-securing moment.

For their part, many therapists are inclined, when a ground rule happens to be secured and their own existential death anxieties are mobilized, to shift to a more cognitive, non-dynamic level of therapeutic work and to find conscious rationalizations that prompt them to undo the frame-securing effort. As humans, we seem to be convinced unconsciously that we cannot cope with the existential death anxieties that secured frames arouse—that they will be the death of us even as their working through can heal our death-related psychic wounds. The fear of death and the existential and predator death anxieties that they evoke are the undoing of many a psychotherapy and human life, and they pose a major threat to all kinds of efforts to gain inner emotional peace, be it in a managed care setting or elsewhere.

AN ILLUSTRATIVE VIGNETTE

In this connection, a clinical vignette reported to me by a male supervisee, Dr. Fuller, comes to mind. He had seen Ms. Young, a thirty-year-old single woman suffering from anxiety attacks, in managed care therapy for about six months when she unexpectedly missed a session. Dr. Fuller decided to keep the patient's time open and to not call her to clarify the basis for her absence. In the consultation session, he had spelled out his patient's responsibility for the fee for last-minute and unannounced absences, explaining that the insurance company did not pay for services not rendered.

Ms. Young came in for her next session and explained that her best friend had been given two free airline tickets to Florida and had asked her to join her for a few days away—and the patient had agreed to go. She was too rushed to call the therapist, to whom she now apologized for not calling or showing up for her session.

The patient went on to talk about the vacation and how impossible it is to meet a good man. While she was away she had a dream in which she was pursuing a man named Ted with whom she had lived for a while when she was in her early twenties. She had a gun in her hand and she cornered him at the end of an alley, stole his wallet, and killed him.

Associating to the dream, she recalled that Ted was a very responsible guy. He had paid the rent for their apartment and for a lot of their daily needs. She owed him a lot of money but had never paid him back; to this day she feels like a thief for not settling her debt. She broke up with him because he was too pushy and demanding; he was right about a lot of the issues that came up between them but she still felt he did not give her room to breathe. She cheated on him by having an affair with an office-mate and when he found out about it, he broke up the relationship.

Changing subjects, Ms. Young recalled a story in a Florida newspaper in which a woman prostitute and her friend had shot and killed one of the men she had slept with; they had murdered then robbed him of his money. Ms. Young could hardly afford to pay her share of the hotel room down there, but she didn't back down from her responsibility to her friend who had so generously paid for her trip. It was the right thing to do and she did it.

Using the adaptive approach, Dr. Fuller asked the patient to go over the themes in her dream and guided associations and to find their connection to what was happening in the therapy situation. Ms. Young could see that she was talking about men and mayhem, but little else. Dr. Fuller pointed to the themes of robbery, murder, and keeping to financial obligations. The patient acknowledged that this must be connected to the fee for her missed session. It prompted her to recall that she wanted to ask her therapist to bill the insurance company for the session; she would back him up on any question they might raise and would give him her co-pay.

Dr. Fuller pointed out that her themes spoke for a very different way of handling the fee for the missed session, which, as she knew, her insurance did not cover. In her dream, she murders and robs a man with whom she had a close relationship, a man she betrayed by having an affair with another man. In proposing to not pay the full fee for the missed session, her unconscious view is that she'd be murdering and robbing the therapist of the money that is his due. In addition, in suggesting that he falsely bill the insurance company for the session, she would be asking him to join her in doing violence to and robbing them of money that neither he nor the patient deserved to have. A look at the themes from her unconscious mind points to the need for her to take full responsibility for the missed session, which she views as her having betrayed the therapist by illicitly and unfaithfully going off with someone else.

Ms. Young paused and then said the dream now reminded her of a time when she had asked Ted to buy some make-up for her and when he did it, she had never paid him the money he had spent. That was downright robbery. All right, she added, she'll pay the full fee—how much is it?

After the therapist told her what the insurance company pays for the patient's session, the patient squirmed a little and complained that the therapist's office was too hot; she could hardly breathe and was beginning to feel anxious. Dr. Fuller linked these feelings to her dream, pointing out that with the frame secured, she seemed to feel cornered and to have become fearful that he would murder her. The patient responded by saying that she did have a pattern of running away from men when her relationship with them became serious, too tight. She then had an image of being buried alive in a coffin and laughed because she could see what it meant—that in taking full responsibility for the missed session she was feeling entrapped and on the verge of being annihilated.

With that the session ended.

This is a vignette that involves an archetypal frame-securing moment. Even when a managed care therapist carefully defines the ground rule related to the patient's responsibility to pay the full fee for missed sessions, patients generally obliterate or repress what they have been told. This is a reflection of their unconsciously motivated, conscious need for modified frames and in addition, an indication of the extent to which they believe on some level that managed care psychotherapy is a frame-modified offer of entitlement that they can abuse as much as they like. For example, most managed care patients who abruptly terminate their therapy will not mail their therapists any unpaid amounts due to them. The unconsciously driven, conscious expectations of a free ride pervades this treatment form.

Yet, as we see here, patients' deep unconscious minds are well aware of the stated ground rule of responsibility for the fee for unannounced missed sessions. In fact, even if the therapist had not articulated this ground rule or had indicated that he would excuse the patient from such a responsibility, on the deep unconscious level of experience and need, the patient nonetheless would have encoded a directive to the therapist to charge her in full for the missed session. Based on in-built, evolved archetypes, this part of her mind knows full well that doing so would support the ideal frame she needed for soundly coping with and insightfully resolving her emotion-related symptoms—patients the world over encode directives of this kind. This point deserves emphasis because many conscious-system psychotherapists naively and erroneously believe that they can offer their patients any set of ground rule they choose and that these rules will work well for the therapy. This is a treacherous conscious-system conviction that does not find support deep unconsciously where universal ground rule precepts hold sway.

Because he is an adaptive psychotherapist, Dr. Fuller had spelled out the ground rule at issue here in the first session with the patient. Even so, because she was beset with her own secured-frame death anxieties (when she was eight, Ms. Young's father had died in a fire), the patient had repressed it consciously—but not deep unconsciously. Consciously, the patient expected to have no responsibility for the fee for the session she missed and thus anticipated that she would be spared the conscious experience of her entrapping, secured-frame, existential death anxieties and their roots in the early life trauma she had suffered.

In typical fashion, the patient, who is not a psychopath, went so far as to try to defend herself against these anxieties by suggesting that the therapist lie to and exploit the insurance company—something that all too many managed care therapists actually do under similar circumstances. This is a conscious invitation to act immorally and to violate the contract with the insurer as well as the law of the land. Were the therapist to do so, he would be unconsciously sanctioning the patient's turn to an immoral and blatantly dishonest frame violation. He thereby unwittingly would be encouraging the patient to act dishonestly and immorally whenever her existential death anxieties were activated. This kind of consequence for a violation of a managed care contract is seldom recognized as such by either party to therapy even though it has devastating unconsciously mediated effects on all concerned.

We can see too that the patient's deep unconscious needs and expectations were the very opposite of their conscious counterparts. On the deep unconscious level of experience, based on the pristine wisdom and morality of its subsystems, Ms. Young knew that she should be held responsible for the full fee for the missed session. This expectation is reflected in the money-related themes that she generated in the session, themes that are replete with *correctives or models of rectification* that even a non-adaptive psychotherapist could use in intervening in regard to a frame issue of this kind.

The vignette also amply illustrates the entrapping, secured-frame, existential death anxieties that the patient experienced in anticipation of the therapist's frame-securing intervention. The therapist's implicit encouragement that the patient report her dreams and associate to them in her sessions helped Ms. Young to express these anxieties in a disguised form that allowed for their trigger decoded interpretation and for a proper frame-management response by the therapist as well. Conscious system psychotherapists tend to manage the ground rules on the basis of their own conscious preferences, which are imposed on their patients in ways that are experienced deep unconsciously as assaultive and predatory. Should a frame-securing moment arrive inadvertently and go uninterpreted, the patient is likely to flee treatment even though his or her secured-frame, existential death anxieties are experienced unconsciously. Patients will make thin conscious excuses for leaving treatment while the unconscious motivating cause for their departure eludes their own and their therapists' conscious appreciation.

The entire scenario is very different when a therapist has narrative themes to interpret and to use as the patient's directives for his or her frame-management efforts. In these cases, the patient is able to see that the therapist is making use of the patient's own deep unconscious needs, insights, and models of rectification, and that the therapist is intervening with the patient's best interests and emotional healing in mind. Frame-securing moments offer patients unique opportunities to experience and adaptively reprocess their deep unconscious existential death anxieties, their sources in death-related traumas, and their adverse effects on their lives. Even so, they are moments of great dread and anxiety for both patient and therapist, and they need to be handled with great sensitivity, optimally by using the patient's narrative imagery as the guide to intervening.

THE EFFECTS OF MODIFIED FRAMES

Frame-modified forms of therapy are inherently predatory of patients because they are exploitative and seductive; they also interfere with the establishment of clear and safe boundaries between the parties to treatment. This basic mode of therapy evokes a patient's deep unconscious (and on occasion, conscious) sense of mistrust and uncertainty regarding the intentions of the frame-breaking therapist. Every departure from the ideal psychotherapy frame is experienced deep unconsciously by both the perpetrator (most often the therapist) and the recipient (most often the patient) as personally harmful and as causing damage to their conjoint efforts to bring well-grounded, lasting emotional relief to the patient. When uncalled-for frame modifications are invoked, the patient is likely to accept them consciously, but he or she also will suffer from severe bouts of unconscious predatory death anxiety based on the deep unconscious experience of being violated and seriously harmed by the therapist. Meanwhile the offending therapist unconsciously sees himself or herself as predating the patient and experiences deep unconscious predator death anxiety and guilt, which is transformed into active, unconsciously driven needs for both reparation and self-punishment—mainly the latter; the therapist unwittingly suffers accordingly.

The potential saving grace for those who must deal with the mandated deviant-frame forms of managed care psychotherapy lies with the aforementioned ability of therapists to hold fast to those ground rules that can be kept secured, and the corresponding commitment of their patients to accept and keep to this minimally compromised set of conditions without seeking further frame modifications. In addition, these potentially adverse effects are lessened by patients' deep unconscious appreciation of their absolute necessity and therapeutically, by therapists using their patients' narrative material to work through and resolve as much as possible the negative consequences of the existing frame deviations on both parties to treatment. Private self-processing efforts by the therapists also can help them to gain some in-depth perspectives on the untoward effects that they are experiencing deep unconsciously because they are working under deviant managed care conditions. For therapists in general, doing psychotherapy under managed care conditions is traumatic and at times, daunting. Ignoring the impact of the prevailing frame modifications on themselves greatly amplifies the damage they cause to all concerned and can render the psychotherapy experience quite tenuous and easily disrupted by the patient.

Because a frame alteration is an action, deviant-frame psychotherapies run the risk of unwittingly promoting harmful forms of acting out by both patients and therapists within and outside of the treatment experience. These costly, maladaptive ways of coping cause damage to all concerned. They are invoked in order to deny death and cope with activated death anxieties in frame-deviant ways that lead to suffering on their part and in those with whom they are close. Turning to frame violations can become a way of life for the patient and a way of both doing therapy and living his or her life for the therapist. Both patients and therapists need to be mindful of the enormity of the effects of the therapeutic environment on the treatment experience and, by natural extension, on their personal lives.

CONSCIOUS ATTITUDES TOWARD FRAMES

It is relatively easy for the human mind to imagine the evolution of a limb or a brain, but quite difficult to imagine minds evolving even though they have done so over millions of years. Given that the inexorable process of natural selection tends to favor the reproduction of organisms with adaptive attributes and systems that enhance survival, the question arises as to why this process has been so partial to conscious minds that deny as many painful, emotionally charged realities and their most anxiety-provoking meanings as possible. In this connection, we also must ask why so many humans prefer consciously to live their lives, and to receive and offer psychotherapy, under conditions that, upon close conscious examination, appear to be patently harmful to their emotional health—to which is added a grim and jaundiced deep unconscious view of the situation.

Some of the problem lies with the natural tendencies of conscious minds, be they of patients or therapists, to ignore frame conditions; to seldom think about the consequences of behaviors that extend beyond appropriate boundaries; and to be all too ready to excuse frame violations with one or another rationalization. This is part of the conscious system's defensive, denial-based approach to life and its traumatizing triggers, and there are two major forces behind these self-defeating attitudes, each worthy of a fresh examination.

The first force is existential death anxiety. Secured frames evoke these, our most dreaded anxieties, while modified frame diffuse or enable us to deny these anxieties, albeit at the price of harm to oneself and others. Based on the unconscious illusion or delusion that a successful frame-breaker is an exception to all of nature's rules, including the existential rule that death follows life, humans generally prefer to interact within modified rather than secured frames. Patients do so for the added reason that they would rather deal with predatory death anxiety than the more dreaded existential form—as noted, they unconsciously realize that they may defeat a predator but cannot in the long run defeat death. Given that existential death anxiety is an inevitable part of life, the best they can do—and they have little faith in this regard—is to develop the adaptive capacity to deal with the inevitability of death in creative and constructive ways that neutralize its potentially detrimental effects.

For their part, rather than endure their own existential death anxieties, therapists unknowingly prefer to suffer from the predator death anxieties and deep unconscious guilt and need for punishment caused by their modifying the archetypal ground rules of therapy far more than the necessary minimum. In this case, predator death anxiety allows for the hope of suffering enough to assuage deep unconscious needs for punishment so as to be set free from one's guilt-ridden need to suffer. There also is the possibility of atonement and reparation, through which a person can gain inner, deep unconscious forgiveness for the harm caused to others. It is then the feeling of ultimate helplessness that makes existential death anxiety the most affecting horror of life on earth and prompts patients and therapists alike to choose frames and behave in ways that evoke predatory and predator death anxiety in lieu of—and as protection against—the existential form.

We pay an enormous price for the evolved, human bias towards frame violating choices because they entail behaviors and decisions that constitute an enacted form of denial that brings with it a false sense of momentary relief but eventually causes harm to all concerned. This preference for frame modifications is an unconscious, inner motivating force that continuously threatens the integrity of the managed care treatment process and it undermines the pursuit of truly adaptive, deeply insightful symptom alleviation. In lieu of insight, frame modifications become a basic way of coping for both patient and therapist, leading to all kinds of ultimately destructive decisions and behaviors. Here too we need to be reminded that unconscious influences, whether consciously recognized or not, have enormously powerful effects on our behavior and lives.

The natural bent for deviant frames in psychotherapy is so strong that most therapists and patients invoke a frame modification whenever it presents itself as a possibility. They rationalize and offer spurious reasons for its invocation and then support their actions with an array of additional denials—for example, that a particular unneeded frame modification is absolutely necessary; that it is of little or no consequence; that the frame violation is not really a frame break; that a patient's symptomatic regression or a therapist's emotional difficulties have nothing to do with the recent frame alteration that actually has evoked it; that secured frames are unnecessarily rigid and antitherapeutic (which they are not); and similar untenable justifications. This denial also may be buttressed by not affording frame conditions the attention they deserve or by working over frame related interventions manifestly and simplistically.

The secured-frame existential death anxieties of both patients and therapists lead them unwittingly into unholy alliances—*misalliances*, as they are termed—in which each party supports the other's costly and damaging needs for frame modifications. By and large, it takes a blatant, grossly destructive frame violation, like a therapist's failing to appear for several sessions or his or her repeatedly canceling hours at the last minute, for the conscious mind of a patient to see that a harmful frame violation has taken place and that it is detrimental to his or her emotional health. Even then, however, most patients will stay with the offending therapist for what is likely to be more of the same. Given that managed care frames depart from the archetypal ideal and are basically modified, and that frame violations beget further frame violations, these problems are especially severe in this form of psychotherapy. Therapists need to be on the alert for their own inclinations to add unneeded frame modifications to these treatment situations and they also should be on the alert for their patients' tendencies to behave in similar fashion.

The second main reason why patients tolerate so much frame-violating abuse from their therapists is to be found in the conscious mind's vulnerability to the effects of deep unconscious guilt for having harmed others, including the resultant unconscious need for punishment by oneself or others. Who among us has not hurt others, both psychologically and, in some instances, physically? The deep unconscious system of morality and ethics demands its "pound of flesh" for these "crimes" and it seizes and creates every possible opportunity to get its due. This devastating unconsciously driven need is fulfilled in the managed care psychotherapy situation when therapists unduly harm their patients through unnecessary frame violations and patients behave towards their therapist in similarly abusive, frame-violating ways. Because these effects are deep unconsciously mediated, they are all but impossible to detect without turning to trigger decoding. Therapists who do not use this method of listening and intervening are well advised to keep as much of the managed care frame intact and secured as possible.

Another serious consequence of being part of a therapy that is unnecessarily frame modified is that both the perpetrator and victim of the frame violation soon take to violating frames in their daily lives and to unnecessarily suffering frame-violating indignities as well. Many managed care therapists who believe that they are working to enable their patients to insightfully modify their emotional ills actually are unwittingly repeating and reinforcing these ills by creating a version of the patient's pathology-promoting, traumatic life experiences at the hands of prior harmful frame violators and their frame violations. Were it not for patients' tendencies to consciously over-idealize their therapists and their therapies and to deny all but the most severe harm therapists do to them, and were it not for the paradoxical ability of humans to, at times, function better rather than worse in response to traumas and hurts, therapists would have cleaned up their uncalled-for frame-deviant acts long ago.

DEEP UNCONSCIOUS ATTITUDES TOWARD FRAMES

All in all, we see again see that we must turn to the far more consistent, wiser, and healing-oriented deep unconscious mind for guidance regarding the ground rules of managed care psychotherapy and for insights into the consequences of therapists' frame-securing and frame-modifying interventions. The deep unconscious system is intensely concerned with the effects of the conditions under which we live, work, and participate in psychotherapy. And it keeps a sharp, steady, albeit unconscious eye on the wisdom and healing values of our frame-related decisions and on the death-related and moral and ethical aspects of how therapists and patients handle and respond to ground-rule conditions.

Deep unconscious attitudes toward frames are of an entirely different order from those that are conscious. While conscious views vary greatly—one therapist's ground rule is another therapist's frame violation—deep unconscious preferences are shared by all humans and, as noted, they consistently speak for and favor an ideal, archetypal, healing secured frame. I have stressed this universal aspect of deep unconscious experience because it is so alien to the conscious-system thinking on which present-day psychoanalysis, psychoanalytically oriented, and less dynamic forms of therapy are based.

As for the adaptive wisdom of frame-related interventions, the deep unconscious system sees and encodes many therapeutic advantages to frame-securing efforts by therapists and when feasible, by their patients. The healing qualities of secured ground rules are enormous and in some forms of private psychotherapy they account for almost all of the curative powers of the therapeutic experience—to the benefit of both parties to treatment. Interpersonally, secured frames evoke a sense of trust, respect, safety, strength in the therapist, his or her empathic attunement with the patient, and similar positive experiences. Secured frames thereby inherently give patients the underlying strength and ego and superego enhancements that facilitate their dealing with their existential death anxieties and other emotional issues, most of them arising as a result of the therapist's handling of the ground rules of treatment. We are reminded that, in principle, triggers—most of them constituted as therapists' interventions, especially those that are frame-related—are the activators of the significant anxieties, conflicts, and the like that patients work through and resolve in treatment. Patients' experiences in psychotherapy basically do not arise from within their minds, that is, from isolated, inner-directed needs that are projected into the therapist and the therapeutic arena. The most significant experiences in psychotherapy involve adaptive responses to anxiety-provoking triggering events, positive or negative in nature. It is these interventional incidents that arouse patients' inner needs and anxieties, which then can be traced to earlier death-related traumatic events that aroused similar issues in the past; unresolved residuals of earlier traumas can thereby be processed and adaptively resolved.

In regard to death and death anxiety, the deep unconscious mind fully appreciates that these anxieties are the fundamental causes of emotional maladaptations and of much of human creativity as well. The system accurately perceives and experiences the death anxieties evoked by countless interventions made by therapists regarding which the conscious mind finds no such issue. Death anxiety most often is experienced outside of awareness and is reflected in death-denying behaviors and, most critically, in the scattered encoded images generated by patients in psychotherapy when these anxieties are activated by a death-related triggering event. These triggers evoke displaced and disguised themes related to death and the key to understanding their unconsciously experienced meanings lies with linking the themes to their evocative triggers. Therapeutic work of this kind reveals that unconscious expressions of death anxiety reflecting each of its basic types—predatory, existential, or predator—are a continuous aspect of human life and that they pervade the psychotherapy situation as well.

Death anxiety is not only a response to unconsciously perceived death-related triggering events, it also is the motivating force behind the turn to unneeded frame violations. *Existential death anxiety* motivates frame modifications as a way of escaping the entrapping qualities of secured frames; *predatory death anxiety* motivates frame violations that are in the service of self-defense and of attempts to harm a threatening, predatory enemy; and *predator death anxiety* prompts the turn to frame violations as a way of provoking others into responding punitively to the guilt-ridden frame violator. This last cause of frame modifications is seen with therapists who modify frames in unconscious attempts to have their patients attack and punish them for harm that they have caused others—or the patient—in the past.

In regard to issues of ethics and morality, patients rarely consciously recognize or think about the moral aspects of a therapist's handling of ground rules and they tend to ignore or deny the ethical issues raised by frame-related interventions. On rare occasions, as seen when a frame violation is grossly dishonest—for example, a therapist submits an inflated bill to an insurer—there may be a conscious ethical assessment by the patient. But more often than not, the therapist's dishonesty is ignored or excused consciously, as is the inevitable harm that such an act brings to everyone involved in the deception. In addition, the more lasting negative effects of this kind of immoral act are subjected to denial even though they involve unconsciously driven self-punitive choices and behaviors.

The deep unconscious mind functions as the guardian of sound morality and ethics. Consistently and with great perceptiveness, the system assesses the moral implications of frame-related activities and fully appreciates—and encodes—the ethical aspects of holding to the ideal frame and the unethical and immoral qualities of frame violations. And this holds true, but in attenuated form, for the mandated frame modification of managed care therapies because patients have a deep unconscious perspective on their necessity.

All in all, then, there is no escaping the deep unconscious effects of the therapeutic environment, be it secured or modified. These ever-present effects should be recognized through trigger decoding and dealt with accordingly. Similarly, unconscious directives to secure aspects of managed care ground rules should be harvested through trigger decoding and whenever possible, followed down to the last detail. I repeat again that the matchless wisdom and pristine morality of the deep unconscious mind is our greatest resource in learning how to conduct effective psychotherapy, how to frame the best possible managed care treatment experience, and how to enable both patients and their therapists to best live their lives.

Chapter Five

The Ground Rules of Managed Care Psychotherapy

I turn now to the many specific issues that arise in connection with the framework of managed care psychotherapy and their effects on all concerned—patients, providers, and insurers. This socially and financially necessitated form of treatment takes place in a therapeutic environment that is neither natural, neutral, nor ideal for the healing of emotion-related problems. Its frame has two very different basic qualities: On the one hand, it is contaminated and endangering, but on the other, under the right circumstances, it can be a situation where these contaminations may be well controlled, only minimally disruptive, and the source of therapeutic insight and healing.

At present, we have no viable means of clearly defining the therapeutic limitations that are, in general, the result of the conditions that prevail in managed care treatment situations. The best that can be said of the situation is that with sound techniques deep healing is feasible under these conditions, and with it, there can be effective symptom alleviation. This is especially the case with an open-ended treatment setting and less so when an insurer sets limits on the number of sessions it will cover for a given patient—overall or in a given year. A forced termination provoked by limitations in a patient's insurance coverage tends to undo much of the healing previously accomplished. It also forces the patient to consider the difficult matter of shifting to private therapy, a choice most patients are loathe to make—they only rarely do so.

In sum, then, it is possible to do effective, symptom-alleviating therapeutic work within the managed care frame, but unique limitations, psychological and practical, may interfere with achieving that goal. As a result, it may well be that managed care patients receive far more pharmacological help than the average private patient.

In practice, the framework offered to a managed care patient is likely to—or should—entail a mixture of secured and modified ground rules. There are a notable number of ground rules that can be installed and sustained in this form of treatment, thereby offering patients—and their therapists—a limited but significant amount of safety, security, and inherently frame-related healing. Their use also speaks for a therapist's moral and ethical integrity and implicitly indicates that he or she has come to terms with his or her death-related issues and anxieties—a resolution that is the *sine qua non* for sound and effective frame management efforts. Indeed, when therapists are in the throes of a current death-related trauma in their personal or professional lives, they are unconsciously driven to modify the ground rules of the treatment experiences whose frames they are managing. There are no barriers between a therapist's personal life and his or her work as a psychotherapist.

SECURABLE GROUND RULES

The ground rules that usually can be secured for a managed care psychotherapy include:

A professional or otherwise uncontaminated referral, with no prior contact between patient and therapist.

The use of a private, professional office setting with a soundproofed office used solely by the therapist.

The therapist as the sole person to have direct therapeutic contact with the patient from the beginning to the end of the treatment.

A set fee structure.

Unvarying arrangements in respect to the time, length, and frequency of sessions.

The therapist's presence at all scheduled sessions.

The patient's requirement to appear for all scheduled sessions and his or her responsibility for the full fee for missed sessions. (This rule may run counter to the policy of some insurance companies; see chapter six.)

A reasonable vacation policy on the part of the therapist.

The relatively anonymity of the therapist.

The use of the basic rule of patients' free associating, supplemented by the rule of guided associations.

The therapist's utilization of neutral interventions.

The absence of physical contact between patient and therapist.

The confinement of contacts between patient and therapist to the time and place of regularly scheduled sessions.

The responsibility for establishing these naturally supportive, constructive, and inherently curative set of ground rules lies primarily with the therapist, but it also requires the understanding of, and acceptance by, the patient.

Acceptance of a secured ground rule is not a natural inclination of the conscious mind so the existence of mandated frame deviations unwittingly encourages patients to seek additional frame modifications. As a result, with therapists who invoke these tenets, it is not unusual for patients to object consciously to their invocation. Among the ground rules that most often become contentious are paying for missed sessions, adhering to the scheduled time for sessions, and accepting the precept that, with some inescapable exceptions, the therapist will not have contact with third parties other than the insurer. Lest the therapist seem arbitrary in invoking and maintaining these ground rules, the use of trigger decoding that reveals the patient's own deep unconscious need for and insistence on these ground rules makes clear the necessity of these frame-securing measures.

As I have indicated, there is a great need in managed care psychotherapy to maintain a secured sector of ground rules that can counterbalance and help to neutralize the negative effects of the mandated frame deviations under which treatment must transpire. These securable ground rules must be given serious consideration by all therapists no matter how they conduct a managed care therapy; they are vital to the lasting, insightful cure of the patient's emotional ills. The unconscious experience of a segment of trust and safety is highly ameliorative for the patient and provides genuine, deep satisfactions for the therapist—and spares him or her a great deal of deep unconscious guilt and its painful consequences.

MANDATED FRAME DEVIATIONS

There are as well a group of inter-related archetypal ground rules that by and large cannot be invoked by managed care therapists because their modification is mandated by the two basic contracts at hand: One between the insurer and the patient and the other between the insurer and the provider. These departures from the ideal frame render all forms of managed care treatment as deviant-frame psychotherapies and they include *the absence of*:

Responsibility for both parties to be present and fiscally responsible for all scheduled sessions. (As noted above, therapists nevertheless may choose to invoke this ground rule.)

Patients' sole responsibility for their therapists' full fee for all scheduled sessions—that is, the absence of third-party payers.

Patients' responsibility to pay their therapists' their fair and accustomed fee for services.

The total privacy and confidentiality of the psychotherapy experience.

The therapist's total therapeutic commitment to the patient and a similar commitment by the patient.

And in some cases the relative anonymity of the therapist, which may be compromised by information provided by the insurance company.

This list pertains solely to the ground rule modifications that are required by most managed care insurers. Many therapists will freely alter other archetypal ground rules in working with their managed care patients largely because they do this with most or all of their patients regardless of the conditions under which they are seen. Representative of these frequently modified ground rules are alterations—both increases, and more rarely, decreases—in the therapist's fee; changes in the time or day of individual sessions; extensions or reductions of the length of sessions; deliberate personal and other self-revelations and advice-giving by the therapist; and a variety of uncalled-for breaches of the privacy and confidentiality of the therapy. All of these deviations are manifestations of the costly human conscious need for deviant frames.

THE EFFECTS OF THE DEVIANT MANAGED CARE FRAME

While the list of unfeasible ground rules is smaller than those that are feasible, it is quite clear that these unavoidable violations of the ideal, unconsciously sought framework for psychotherapy have considerable impact and extensive consequences for managed care patients and their therapists—and for the insurers who sponsor their therapeutic interactions. The effects of these deviations fall into two classes: Those that are shared by all frame-deviations and those that are specific to the particular frame modification that has been invoked.

The effects of both of these factors on patients and therapists tend to be universal—that is, everyone is affected in similar fashion by the deviant conditions of treatment. Individual factors come into play mainly in respect to a given patient's or therapist's sensitivity to, and capacity to cope with, particular universal meanings to which they are especially vulnerable. Most of these selective sensitivities arise from the patient's previous experiences with secured and modified frames and the history of their death-related traumas. Of note in this regard is the finding that prior frame-violating experiences create opposing unconscious needs: On the one hand, the need for further denial-promoting deviant frames; on the other, a need for for safe, secured frames. Most often, but by no means always, the turn to frame modifications prevails.

Many overly traumatized patients are extremely sensitive to the harm caused by frame violations, but much of this is experienced and conveyed unconsciously rather than consciously. For example, some patients who have been illicitly abused sexually by parental figures or whose parents have created publicly exposed scandals are especially affected by the absence of full privacy and confidentiality. Others with comparable histories of sexual abuse will yearn unconsciously for a secured frame. Nevertheless, these patients often are consciously inclined to seek frame modifications because they are afraid that the secured frame will be more entrapping than safe and that they will be abused in some sexual or non-sexual way by their therapists—that is, that as in their childhoods, the promise of a secured frame will be betrayed.

Another paradox inherent to the compromised managed care frame lies with the finding that on the one hand, the frame itself causes harm to patients (and their therapists), while on the other, it presents patients with an extraordinary opportunity to work through their predatory death anxieties and their prior experience of frame violations earlier in their lives. This is possible, however, only if the frame modification is not severely toxic and is properly interpreted through trigger decoding—and rectified if possible. Under these conditions the healing effects outdo the harm involved.

SOME THERAPEUTIC PRINCIPLES

Insightful therapeutic relief and change are, as noted, quite possible under managed care conditions. The outcome depends on a variety of factors such as those that pertain to the therapist's management of the remainder of the therapeutic framework, the patient's emotion-related history and especially his or her history of death-related and frame-related traumas, patients' conscious frame inclinations, the extent to which the therapist pays attention to the framework of treatment, and the nature of the other components of the therapeutic work carried out by the therapist. Given the multiplicity of factors, the outcome of these treatment experiences tends to vary greatly from one patient to the next. In principle, then, insight-oriented and other forms of emotional healing are afforded full support when a therapist is able to adopt the following frame-related measures:

Secures those parts of the frame that are not affected by the provider's mandated frame modifications.

Keeps the mandated frame violations to an absolute minimum.

Avoids adding unneeded frame modifications to those that are absolutely necessary.

Keeps the frame as stable as possible and responds in a frame-securing manner to a patient's requests for frame modifications, basing his or her interventions as much as possible on trigger decoding the patient's narrative images.

Explores, processes, trigger decodes, and interprets the patient's deep unconscious perceptions and experiences of the ground rule modifications that are framing the therapy, doing so when they are activated by a triggering event relevant to the therapist's management of the frame.

Attempts to rectify a deviant ground rule as conditions permit and the patient's material unconsciously directs.

Traces a patient's current frame-related reactions to his or her past death-related, frame-violating traumas and uses these links to illuminate the largely unconscious sources of the patient's emotional maladaptations—and to thereby enable the patient to resolve the emotionally damaging, unconsciously mediated consequences of these past traumas.

THE GENERAL EFFECTS OF MANAGED CARE FRAME DEVIATIONS

Clinical study using the adaptive approach reveals some surprising trends regarding the general effects of managed care frames. Despite their conscious naiveté and lack of conscious frame-related knowledge, *most patients will, in their initial sessions, encode a negative deep unconscious reaction to one or more of the archetypal frame modifications built into their managed care psychotherapy.* This trend is striking evidence for the universality of the need for an ideal frame. It also indicates that psycho-biologically and by virtue of natural selection and evolutionary processes, the deep unconscious mind has acquired the natural wisdom to appreciate the features of the ideal, curative frame and to know when it is compromised.

The most common frame issues addressed early on are the lack of privacy and confidentiality, the presence of the third-party payer, and the therapist's compromised commitment to the patient. These concerns are not expressed consciously in that, short of an acute, unexpected frame-issue, a patient almost never brings up these frame deviations directly—they are as a rule consciously obliterated and not matters of conscious concern. In addition, when the encoded expression pertaining to these issues is detected and interpreted by the therapist on the basis of trigger decoding the patient's encoded themes, the patient almost always will deny having any conscious concern about the deviations, which they nevertheless are working over deep unconsciously.

This mental split—that is, the ever-present differences between conscious and deep unconscious experiences, concerns, needs, and adaptive strategies—is in evidence during these moments in therapy. Even so, with therapists who have not developed an ear for encoded frame-related themes, the narrative material will be dealt with manifestly without appreciating its deep unconscious meanings. To be understood as such, encoded themes must be met partway by a sensitive ear and most therapists are tone-deaf in this regard—victims of the naïve default position of the conscious mind.

CLINICAL ILLUSTRATIONS

For example, in the consultation session and more often in the following two or three sessions, managed care patients will report dreams and associations, or tell stories about intrusive third parties, treacherous benefactors, public exposure, and the like. Left to their natural inclinations, therapists will not link these images to the frame violations at hand, but will instead try to formulate some kind of psychodynamic, patient-centered, non-interactive meaning from the material.

A typical example was seen in the second session of her managed care psychotherapy with Mr. Albert, a male social worker, when his patient, Mrs. Brown, reported dreaming of a man peeking at her through the window of her bedroom. One of her associations was to a local peeping Tom whose activities were reported in the newspaper: He had entered a couple's bedroom through an open window while they were talking to each other in bed; he then raped the woman and badly beat the man.

Most therapists would formulate this material in terms of the patient's sexual conflicts with men and possibly her husband. This is a formulation with some merit, but it would not obtain encoded confirmation. This non-validation unconsciously would arise because the interpretation avoids and denies the more pertinent connections of this imagery to the therapist and to the mandated frame-deviant triggers for which he is presently responsible.

Mr. Albert, who worked adaptively, intervened by noting that the patient had alluded to a man and woman talking, much as he and the patient were doing at the moment. He proposed that this bridging theme indicated that the dream reflects the patient's unconscious experience of some aspect of the therapy situation. Mrs. Brown drew a blank and the therapist then pointed to the image of a criminal intruder and asked her if there wasn't a third party intruder in her therapy. She responded in the negative but when Mr. Albert challenged her, she thought for a while and then laughed, saying that he couldn't be referring to the insurance company, could he? Even so, she immediately denied that she was at all concerned about the insurer—everything is done with computers these days. But Mr. Albert responded that her imagery indicated that her deep unconscious mind thought otherwise. On that level of experience Mrs. Brown evidently viewed the insurance company as an intrusive third party to her therapy and using her encoded themes, he pointed out that the violation of the boundaries and privacy of her treatment was being experienced as causing violent harm to both herself and him.

The patient responded by saying that she needed the insurance coverage in order to be in therapy. Mr. Albert then asked her to find another incident that the dream brought to mind and Mrs. Brown remembered being in bed with her husband one night three years ago when he suddenly turned to her and guessed that she was pregnant. They had not been trying to have a child but he was right; they were both thrilled about it. Dr. Albert pointed out that this association suggested that unconsciously, she was confirming his intervention, adding that his being on the mark seemed to be viewed by the patient as an opportunity for her to begin a new life. With that, the time was up.

Deciphering patients' deep unconsciously fashioned encoded communications calls for a decoding stance in the therapist. This enables him or her to listen in a way that leads to the development of trigger decoded interpretations and sound efforts at frame securing where feasible. This effort begins as a rule with the identification of the most active and cogent trigger to which the patient is reacting deep unconsciously. With the trigger tentatively identified, the therapist then listens to the patient's narrative images as they form a rebus or scattering of related themes that tell the story of the patient's deep unconscious perceptions and understanding of the triggering event. The therapist attends to these themes to determine if they appear to organize and coalesce around the postulated triggering intervention. This is a method of silent formulation and an attempt at unconscious validation and if it fails, the therapist must revise his or her thinking and, in most instances, seek another triggering event as the main source of the encoded imagery.

This particular vignette is typical of patients' early reactions to the deviant ground rules of managed care psychotherapy. The trigger is not mentioned directly and is of no conscious concern to the patient, who expresses a series of conscious denials in response to her therapist's trigger-decoded interpretations. Nevertheless, the patient's deep unconscious mind appears to be reacting adversely to the deviant ground rules of her therapy and the themes she generated speak for her anxieties regarding the modified boundaries, privacy, and confidentiality of her managed care treatment. The third party is experienced deep unconsciously as a murderous, rapacious intruder who is trying to destroy both the patient and the therapist—and to derail the therapy as well.

If the damage caused by managed care frame violations goes uninterpreted and continues to disturb the patient deep unconsciously, he or she may end the therapy because of the harm that is being experienced deep unconsciously even though the definitive reasons for doing so are unknown to either party to the therapy. On the other hand, the adaptive therapist who trigger decodes and interprets these damaging, frame-related, deep unconscious perceptions usually finds that this therapeutic work enables the patient, who has encoded these concerns, to become consciously aware of these issues in a convincing manner and thereby remain in therapy, experience a healing moment, and continue his or her pursuit of deep insight and emotional relief.

As noted, barring an acute situation that re-ignites concerns about the modified frame conditions, in an adaptive form of psychotherapy the patient's deep unconscious anxieties about the adverse effects of the required managed care frame violations tend to recede into the background and the encoded themes no longer touch on this issue. Instead, other triggers come to the fore and they serve as the prime movers of the patient's imagery and deep unconscious experiences. These triggers tend to activate the early- and later-life traumas that are the sources of the patient's emotional dysfunctions. The working through of these issues takes a fair amount of time but such therapeutic work can indeed eventually lead to a deeply insightful cure.

A note of caution: Patients with a history of severe death-related traumas tend to unconsciously dread the activation of these traumas. They also intuitively realize that therapists who make use of trigger decoding also tend to secure the ideal psychotherapy frame available under the prevailing conditions. Many of these patients therefore are fearful of the deep unconscious death anxieties that the optimal frame will evoke in them and they also are afraid of, and tend to blot out, the encoded narrative imagery that tells in disguise the story of their early traumas and their consequences. Their dread of deep unconscious experience is so intense that they may abruptly terminate their adaptive psychotherapy at the time of the first trigger-decoded interpretation or frame-securing moment. With these patients, a therapist often is damned if he does offer trigger decoded interpretations related to these horrendous issues and damned if he doesn't do so because he or she is then viewed unconsciously as being afraid of these traumas and thus of no use to the patient.

Along different lines, many disruptive moments in managed care psychotherapy arise in response to therapists' unexplored modifications of one or more of the ground rules of therapy, including frame breaks that extend a mandated deviant ground rule. For example, when a therapist makes a frame-violating personal revelation to a patient, scattered themes of exposure, inappropriate nudity, and the like will appear; they need to be heard and decoded for what they are on the encoded level of communication. Failure to do so means that the deviant act will go uninterpreted and unrecognized consciously, paving the way for further harmful self-revelations and other frame modifications that may, at times, overwhelm the patient's psyche. The outcome often is what seems to a manifest-content therapist to be an inexplicable shift to intractable resistances and even the unexpected decision to terminate treatment. A similar dilemma can occur when a therapist, with the patient's permission and full conscious support, tenders a report to an insurance company. Encoded themes of betrayal, divided loyalties, making damaging secrets public, and the like will appear in the narrative imagery and pose a problem not unlike the one just detailed.

The deep unconscious response to a triggering intervention is always present—it is an evolved psychobiological reaction. The problem lies with whether a therapist hears and understands the encoded meanings of the themes at hand.

Typically, patients tend to respond to the invocation of a deviant ground rule with adverse developments such as an intensification of his or her emotional symptoms or interpersonal difficulties. Severe resistances against the therapeutic process and expressions of vague complaints against the therapist also are not uncommon. Many premature terminations of treatment arise on this basis and, quite importantly, unrecognized frame modifications is one of the most common reasons that a therapist feels puzzled and frustrated with his or her patient's failure to improve clinically. This situation also is a common cause of therapists' decisions to turn to the use of psychotropic medications.

All in all, the failure to appreciate and work through the frame-modified conditions of managed care psychotherapy when a patient's deep unconscious mind becomes disturbed by these conditions is one of the most frequent underlying causes of patients' unfavorable responses to treatment. Understanding the deep unconscious sources of these regressions depends on a therapist's sensitivity to the nature and ramifications of the overall managed care frame and to his or her active frame-related interventions—and on being prepared to decode and interpret patients' encoded narrative themes in light of these triggers.

THE PRACTICAL CONSEQUENCES OF MANAGED CARE FRAME DEVIATIONS

The modified frames of managed care psychotherapy have a number of broad, universally negative effects on both patients and therapists, and on the general course of a given psychotherapy experience. Everyone concerned with this type of treatment experience needs to be mindful of these likely disturbances so they can better tolerate them when they materialize and find the means of working them through with the patient in order to turn these traumatic incidents to therapeutic advantage.

It is, of course, difficult to generalize about the features of a so-called average psychotherapy experience. Nevertheless, in trying to characterize the distinctive features of managed care therapy I shall draw on my thirty years as a practitioner with both private and managed care patients. There are some impressive differences between my experiences with patients I've seen within these two treatment frames and clinical evidence suggests that they mainly are a consequence of the modified frames mandated in connection with the managed care situation. Identifying these disruptive effects is the only basis on which we can keep them to a minimum, properly process them, and neutralize their adverse effects.

Some Positive Features

Before delineating the negative side of the managed care situation, I want to make clear again that as long as a therapist restricts himself or herself to the mandated manage care frame modifications, it is quite feasible to conduct the psychotherapy in a manner that produces positive therapeutic results that are more or less comparable to those accomplished in secured, private psychotherapy settings of a comparable duration. Even when the managed care frame is, of necessity, unduly compromised, constructive therapeutic work is feasible, although it is helpful if some of the therapeutic work is directed at the patient's deep unconscious perceptions of the prevailing frame deviations and at efforts at rectification, where possible. Therapists who work on the basis of non-adaptive paradigms of treatment are advised to guard against unnecessary frame modifications and to otherwise conduct their therapies using the same principles they follow in private treatment settings.

The potential for healing in managed care psychotherapy arises because the critical unconscious meanings of patients' core emotional traumas and the emotional problems that these incidents have created for them lie latent and unarticulated until an intervention by their therapist activates the problem area. That is, patients' innermost, death-related, and other secrets and issues lie quiescent until something a therapist says or does—and usually it is frame-related—arouses the relevant unconscious constellations, which then find encoded expression in patients' material; more rarely, the reactivation occurs in response to an extremely damaging outside trauma, like the death of a loved one. With the proper use of trigger decoding and interpretation, fresh insight and healing is likely to materialize. In principle, then, current traumas, most often in the therapy, activate past traumas and bring them to life in the present and into the ongoing work with the therapist—at which time they become available for fresh efforts at resolution.

Implied here is the realization that, since so much depends on the triggers created by the therapist, one set of patients' emotional issues will be activated in secured-frame psychotherapy and quite another set under deviant-frame conditions. Secured-frame reactivations are centered on traumas that have evoked existential and predator death anxieties, while deviant-frame reactivations tend to arouse predatory death anxieties based on past experiences of harm from others and from natural disasters. As noted, in managed care therapies, the predatory features of the mandated deviant frame tend to find expression in sessions that take place early in treatment and then recede into the background unless they are reactivated by an incident that brings up the deviant ground rule—be it triggered by the patient, therapist, or insurer. On the other hand, secured-frame death anxieties arise only when a therapist either secures an aspect of the ground rules or sustains an archetypal rule in the face of a request by the patient to change it. Predator death anxiety and deep unconscious guilt also tend to be activated in secured frames because the secured frame provides a safe space in which the patient can work over residuals of unresolved guilt.

Adaptive forms of psychotherapy are ideally suited to exploring and dealing with these frame issues and the death anxieties that they evoke in both patient and therapist. Engaging in trigger-decoded therapeutic measures carries with it a great deal of damage control in regard to the negative aspects of the deviant managed care frame and facilitates deep unconscious healing.

Some Negative Features

In comparison with private psychotherapy, the inherently frame-modified managed care psychotherapy situation tends to have the following adverse effects, which vary in extent and influence from patient to patient and therapist to therapist. Thus compared to private treatment, managed care therapies tend to be characterized by:

1. A greater amount of frame-related instability caused by the totality of the mandated deviant-frame conditions of treatment. For patients, this instability is manifested through frequent, unexpected cancellations of sessions; failures to appear for consultation sessions with or without notifying the therapist; non-payment of fees that are rightfully due to the therapist; and precipitous, premature terminations of treatment by telephone or by simply not returning for further sessions. On the part of therapists, there tends to be a notable tendency to engage in irresponsible, non-mandated, frame altering behaviors such as beginning sessions late, reducing the agreed-on length of sessions, missing sessions, talking on the telephone during sessions, and similar untoward practices.
2. A reduced commitment to the therapy and a notable measure of mistrust of the other party by both patients and therapists. A notable factor in these attitudes, which tend to exist both consciously and deep unconsciously, is the impersonal, mechanical manner in which patients select their therapists, usually from a list of providers; these inclinations are intensified by the requirement that at times, therapists release patient-related information to insurers. Patients tend to develop paranoid-like attitudes and experience vague or explicit feelings of mistrust and suspiciousness of their therapists. They are inclined to treat their sessions cavalierly as hours they might or might not attend and often give priority to other commitments, some of them quite unimportant, over their commitment to the therapist and therapeutic work. In the extreme, there may be an explicit belief that the therapist is secretly recording sessions or making revelations to unauthorized third parties. In addition, even when a therapist carefully spells out a patient's responsibility to be present for therapy at a given time each week, patients will request changes in this ground rule and even expect that they can modify this tenet at will. For their part, therapists tend to be wary of their patients because of the frequency with which they act out in unexpected ways that are harmful to them, such as suddenly terminating treatment or failing to pay the fees for which they are responsible. Patients' lax approaches

to attendance at sessions may prompt therapists to adopt a similarly lax approach as well. Therapists also react to patients' detachment with similar feelings of their own, and many poorly thought out, unneeded frame violations are invoked as a result.

3. An increase in experiences of deep unconscious—and far more rarely, conscious—guilt in patients because of their deep unconscious tendency to see themselves as responsible for insurers' exploitation of managed care therapists. These felt exploitations include the low overall fee paid to the therapist, the patient being responsible for only a small part of the fee, and the license given to patients to cancel sessions with—and in some cases without—advance notice. Unexplored and unresolved, this guilt can cause patients to behave in ways that are self-punitive and self-harmful—and damaging to the therapeutic process.
4. The greater propensity in both parties to therapy to extend the mandated frame deviations with additional frame violations. Like viruses, frame violations beget frame violations, causing harm to all concerned.
5. For both patients and therapists boundary violations and defiance of ground rules tend more often to become costly but preferred ways of coping with trauma and anxiety, inside and outside of therapy.
6. The more extensive appearance in patients of deep unconsciously driven *gross behavioral resistances* (Langs 1993, 2004) to the therapy that take shape as verbal complaints about the therapist and treatment, uncalled-for absences, and premature terminations of treatment. There is as well a striking amount of *communicative resistances* as seen when patients fail to generate the deep unconsciously based narrative material that usually is conveyed when a frame-related triggering event takes place in the therapy. All in all, then, there are a plethora of gross behavioral and communicative resistances that tend to limit the opportunity for therapeutic intervention and insight.
7. Both consciously and unconsciously patients are more guarded and more inclined to restrict what they reveal about themselves and their emotion-related traumas and anxieties, including their manifest and disguised thoughts and feelings about their therapists. They less often allude directly to active triggers such as a newly modified ground rule and they also tend to limit more the expression of the encoded themes that might otherwise emerge on the basis of their archetypal unconscious perceptions of the universal meanings of such frame modifications. Secrets, kept knowingly and unknowingly, many of them ultimately death-related and critical to understanding the patient's emotional difficulties, also are more commonly kept and the critical links that connect a patient's reactions to an immediate trigger to an earlier death-related trauma also tend to be more sparsely conveyed.

8. It takes considerably more time for managed care patients to encode the expected correctives for those mandated or unnecessary frame deviations that can be rectified in the course of a particular psychotherapy. These *models of rectification* are relatively infrequent and when they do emerge, they tend to be heavily disguised. As a result, accepted frame-securing interventions are relatively uncommon—for example, a shift to private therapy with a patient who can afford to do so. Especially with patients who have suffered from severe past death-related traumas, there is a greater mental set that leads them to expect that existing frame-modifications will continue unabated. The possibility of securing an aspect of the frame and the anticipation of the related existential death anxieties tends more often to unconsciously motivate these patients to disallow and be consciously impervious to their own deep unconscious, encoded frame-securing recommendations. In the face of continuing encoded frame-securing directives, rather than make the positive frame change, the patient is more likely to abruptly terminate the therapy.
9. For a variety of reasons, then, the greater amount of resistances that abound in this treatment modality can make the achievement of the emotion-related relief that the patient seeks an overly long process.
10. Another common problem seen more frequently in the managed care situation arises with overly traumatized patients who have intense fears of deep unconscious meaning because they have fragile egos that are easily overwhelmed by the deep unconscious mind's primitive and grim ways of experiencing traumatic incidents. These patients are inclined to terminate their treatment abruptly at times of severe emotional crises in their daily lives or at a juncture in their therapy when their deep unconscious experiences and issues begin to surface. Without an entirely stable frame to hold them and inherently support their fragile psyches, they tend to take flight far more often than seen with private patients with similar issues.
11. As for therapists who carry out managed care psychotherapy, the modified frame unconsciously motivates them to invoke many more unneeded additional frame violations, most of them highly damaging to both themselves and their patients. They also tend to be lax in dealing with issues related to the deviant conditions of the therapy and because of their own unconscious frame-deviant needs, which are supported by the altered managed care frame, they tend to be especially reluctant, and often miss opportunities, to secure aspects of the frame that lend themselves to such tightening.
12. Along different lines, therapists are generally more frustrated with their work in managed care than they are with private patients. They

are more likely to suffer consciously and deep unconsciously because they are unwittingly predated by the conditions of treatment. They also tend to be frustrated by the relatively strong resistances and erratic behaviors of their patients. In addition, managed care therapists tend to feel demeaned by the fees they receive and by being mandated to engage in frame-deviant practices that do not serve their patients' best interests—or their own. Another common set of unique problems arises because of adverse and antagonistic rulings by insurers, which tend to disturb their work with their patients.

13. Patients' deep unconscious minds tend to have two special, competing perceptions of their managed care psychotherapists. On the one hand, a therapist's decision to do therapy under frame modified conditions is seen as predatory of the patient and unethical. But on the other hand, especially with therapists who sustain the other ground rules of the treatment and work effectively with their patients' material, there is an additional view of the therapist as a well meaning, effective caretaker who is offering patients therapy conditions that make it possible for them to achieve emotion-related healing. In some cases but far less often than seen in private treatment, the positive unconscious view prevails and the therapist becomes available unconsciously to the patient as a source of positive identifications and as a constructive figure whom the patient is able to take in psychologically (introject) in ways that contribute to the curative process.
14. All in all, while the deviant frame contributes to a more unstable and unpredictable treatment situation, it nevertheless is possible to carry out successful insight-oriented and other kinds of psychotherapy under managed care conditions. It seems best to think of this treatment modality as an attenuated form of high-resistance, insecure-frame psychotherapy in which much insight and positive clinical results can be achieved in the face of unique pressures that conspire to undermine the pursuit of insight and the outcome of treatment. The more therapists know about these counter-curative forces, the more likely it is that they will be able to help their patients to resolve or neutralize their adverse effects. Managed care psychotherapy is not a cordial treatment form for overly naïve, denial-prone psychotherapists—or their patients.

In concluding this discussion, it seems clear that managed care psychotherapy does not take place on a level playing field. Instead, the field in which these interactions take place has ill-defined boundaries and ground rules that tend to be arbitrary, uncertain, and changeable. It takes a great deal of skill for therapists to help their patients to be winners under these conditions, but it certainly can be done. To further promote such efforts, I turn now to the specific ground rules of managed care psychotherapy and the particular issues raised by each of them.

Chapter Six

Fee Issues in Managed Care Psychotherapy

In approaching the management of the particular ground rules of managed care psychotherapy and medication management, I turn first to an extensive discussion of the many issues that arise in dealing with the fees that are due to and collected by managed care psychotherapists and psychiatrists. Given the personal investment therapists have in earning a livelihood and the enormous sensitivity of both patients and therapists to money matters, there is little doubt that the handling of fees is one of the most contentious and troublesome issues managed care therapists are called on to deal with. But before presenting my findings and comments, several fresh perspectives on the subject of rules, frames, and boundaries are called for.

TYPES OF FRAME MODIFICATIONS

Because we will be looking into a variety of departures from the archetypal frame, it will be helpful to recognize the four basic types of frame modifications that therapists may initiate in the managed care treatment setting. Each shares in the fundamental effects of frame violations, but each does so with greater or lesser intensity and consequences depending on its nature.

The four classes of frame alterations are:

1. *Frame modifications that are inherent to managed care contracts.*

In principle, these deviations have the usual effects of modified ground rules, but with considerable diminution because of the presence of conscious and unconscious perspectives by both patients and therapists as to their necessity.

2. *Inadvertent frame modifications.*

At times, a therapist will unwittingly further modify the deviant managed care frame without consciously realizing that this is the case. Because the patient will register and be affected by the frame violation deep unconsciously and more rarely notice it consciously, there is need in these instances for the therapist to catch the lapse soon after it has been enacted—and to rectify it if at all possible. Help in doing so is available from the patient because the themes in his or her encoded imagery will bridge over and point to the consciously unrecognized but deep unconsciously experienced frame alteration. While these lapses are persecutory of the patient, if the deviation is not too severe, the naiveté behind the frame lapse tends to limit its negative effects on both parties to the therapy. In some situations, however, these frame violations can have a significant damaging influence on all concerned. An example of this latter type of deviation is seen when a therapist accidentally begins a session late without realizing that he or she has done so. If the deviation is not consciously recognized as such by the therapist and not worked through with the patient on the basis of his or her deep unconscious, encoded narrative material, this kind of frame modification, which is likely to be repeated, can cause considerable harm to all concerned.

3. *Deliberate frame modifications beyond those that are mandated by the managed care contract.*

These frame violations usually are the result of a therapist's lack of familiarity with the deep unconscious level of experience and frame-related archetypes. They may or may not be well meaning, but all too often, they serve the therapist's maladaptive defenses against his or her unresolved death anxieties; they do not satisfy the therapeutic needs of the patient. These deviations evoke three kinds of responses in patients: The usual archetypal reactions to frame deviations; reactions to the specific deviation involved; and personally selective responses that depend on their prior frame-related and death-related experiences and the nature of the modified ground rule.

4. *Deliberate frame modifications that violate the managed care contract.*

These illicit and often illegal frame modifications usually are knowingly invoked by therapists and are, at times, responses to requests from their patients; they always are harmful to both parties to treatment. An example of this type of deviation is that of false billing practices that are corrupt, criminal, immoral, and maladaptive frame violations. Their devastating effects on both patient and therapist may be mediated consciously or unconsciously—more often the latter—and they are the unconscious source of considerable emotional suffering for both parties to treatment. A dishonest therapist cannot honestly heal his or her patients.

ANOTHER PERSPECTIVE

One other basic perspective is needed before looking at the details of the ground rules of managed care psychotherapy and their potential abuses. Each of the frame deviations I shall be discussing causes a measure of harm to both patient and therapist—although unconsciously mediated, each is damaging in very real ways. While the adverse effects of mandated departures from the archetypal frame can be muted because of their necessity, unneeded frame violations tend to cause blatant psychological damage to both parties to treatment. And the more unnecessary and dishonest the frame violation, the greater the harm.

In situations in which the therapist is the prime mover, the damage done to the patient includes an increase in symptoms; justified mistrust of the therapist and, via displacement, others as well; paranoid-like thinking and feelings toward the therapist and others; a preference for harmful frame violations in therapy and in coping with traumas in everyday life; other kinds of damaging forms of acting out against oneself and others, such as attacking or abandoning a significant other without justification—an act that is based on the displacement of rage from the therapist to the outside figure; a justified increase in resistances within the therapy, which interferes with therapeutic progress; anti-therapeutic attacks on the therapist; premature termination of the therapy, which may be a sound coping response to an errant therapist; a mistrust of future therapists and a jaundiced view of psychotherapy; staying with a therapist who is being harmful when termination would be best for the patient; and holding onto destructive relationships outside of treatment—all this and much more.

As for the unnecessarily frame-deviant therapist, the consequences for him or her include the development of predator death anxiety and deep unconscious guilt, which leads to self-harmful, self-punishing decisions and behaviors; the development of psychologically founded symptoms, such as psychosomatic difficulties and untoward experiences of depression and anxiety in the office and everyday life; seemingly inexplicable untoward interpersonal problems professionally and socially; undue disillusionment with the practice and field of psychotherapy; at great cost to self and others, a tendency to turn to frame violations when dealing with stresses within and outside of his or her professional life; a wide variety of irrational and provocative behaviors and beliefs that are expressed in his or her professional relationships and thinking; similarly irrational behaviors in his or her everyday life; all manner of other kinds of interpersonal problems; and sexual and aggressive acting out with patients and others—again, all that and much more.

We can only wonder at the passive process of natural selection that has given form to humans with conscious minds that tolerate or lean towards frame violating behaviors within and outside of the therapy situation that blatantly and subtly cause so much harm to all concerned. But such is one of the grim truths of human nature. That said, in the discussions that follow, I will not reiterate this gruesome and disturbing list of consequences of unnecessary frame violations, even though they bear repetition as fair warning to the many therapists who have accepted the set of unique and heavy responsibilities to patients—and themselves—that come from their distinctive roles as managed care psychotherapists.

With this in mind, let's look now at the vicissitudes of therapists' handling of fees in managed care psychotherapies. We may be forewarned by the biblical phrase "the love of money is the root of all evil," although it would be more to the point to say that "the love of money as it is related to the fear of death is the root of most of the evils seen in the managed care treatment situation" (Langs 2008).

THE ARCHETYPAL FEE-RELATED GROUND RULE

The following is an expanded statement of the unconsciously sought, ideal secured-frame ground rule of psychotherapy as it applies to therapists' fees. I shall use it as the yardstick against which I shall evaluate and discuss managed care fee structures:

Therapists should charge their patients their usual and customary fee for all of their sessions, one that is commensurate with their training and expertise and in keeping with the fee scales that prevail in their community. The fee should be stated by the therapist during the consultation session and not subjected to negotiation. It should apply to all scheduled sessions for which the therapist is available, including the initial "hour" and those sessions that are missed by the patient regardless of the reason. The therapist should handle the fee entirely on his or her own. The fee should be collected on a monthly basis, in that the patient should pay for each month's sessions at the beginning of the first session of the following month. The patient should be responsible for and pay the entire fee by check and the therapist should deposit the check in timely fashion, marking it "for deposit only" to assure its proper disposition. No monthly bill is given to the patient because the check serves as evidence of payment, if needed. Finally, subject to rare exceptions (see below), the fee should remain the same throughout the course of treatment.

THE MANAGED CARE FEE SITUATION

With this in mind, I shall now characterize the essential attributes of the fee arrangements in managed care psychotherapy. By and large, there are two basic situations:

In the first, patients have no co-pay and the insurer covers the therapist's entire fee.

In the second, patients are obligated to pay their therapists a relatively small co-pay for each session. This payment is the same regardless of the duration of the session, which ranges from a fifteen or twenty-minute medication check-up to a one hour psychotherapy visit. The co-pay generally ranges from five to fifty dollars; most are in the fifteen to twenty-five dollar range. The amount varies from one insurer to another and from patient to patient because providers offer contracts to different groups of beneficiaries with fee structures that vary considerably. In all cases, patients' monetary responsibilities for their psychotherapy entail departures from the ideal frame in that they pay their therapists a strikingly small amount of money. Insurers pay the balance of the therapist's fee.

Some insurers mandate that their provider-therapists obtain prior authorization for the consultation and subsequent sessions; an outpatient treatment report also may be required, especially for therapies that extend beyond a few months. These requirements tend to vary depending on the contract between the insurer and the patient as well as by the professional degree earned by the therapist.

Whatever the preliminaries, providers require that payment be based on the submission of a form by mail, fax, or computer. At the very least, it must include a diagnosis, date of service, and the type of service rendered. This information may be provided by the therapist himself or herself, or by a representative such as a secretary or billing service (see below). The time taken by insurance companies to pay their providers ranges from about two to eight weeks, four weeks being the median.

All in all, then, managed payment arrangements are not only basically frame-deviant, they also create a wide range of opportunities for therapists to engage in additional frame modifications that are fully accepted by insurers and most patients. Further confounding the situation, insurers make occasional errors in responding to payment requests. All in all, insurers have a great deal of say and control over the therapies that they sponsor, including their duration and the fees paid to providers.

With few exceptions largely dependent on where a therapist practices, the total fee paid to a therapist is lower than his or her usual, private psychotherapy fee and lower than the fees charged by his or her colleagues for private treatment. This is especially true of psychiatrists who do medication management because in many areas, private fees are extraordinarily high and managed care fees notably low. Along different lines, most insurers maintain a sliding scale of fees that calls for the largest amounts to be paid to psychiatrists, and lesser amounts to psychologists, social workers, and nurse practitioners in some type of descending order.

In most situations, neither the patient nor the insurer is responsible for the fees for sessions canceled by a patient with advance notice—the usual requirement is 24 or 48 hours before the scheduled hour. Insurers also do not pay for services not rendered for any other reason. Under these circumstances, the therapist simply suffers a loss of income. Some therapists believe that they are justified in collecting the co-pay for these sessions from their patients; some insurers would question this position, although others, like Medicare and Medicaid, explicitly forbid therapists to do so. Many therapists will try to use the canceled time for a last-minute consultation with another patient. In severely frame-deviant, dishonest fashion, there also are therapists who collect the co-pay or even the full fee from the patient who canceled his or her session and also accept the consultation fee from another patient seen in their time slot, thereby collecting two fees for the single hour. This type of exploitative frame, deviation is fostered by the inherently deviant managed care frame, which, for both conscious and unconscious reasons, encourages this kind of nevertheless unjustified dishonesty.

In principle, managed care therapists should, as is proper in private therapy, lease a particular segment of time to an ongoing therapy patient; forgiving the patient's fee for a scheduled session for any reason is frame deviant. In situations in which a therapist forgives the fee from an absent patient because he or she has seen another patient in that time slot, the frame for the first patient is still compromised because doing so accepts and sanctions his or her frame-deviant absence and also brings a third party, however shadowy, into the original patient's therapy. This is why the archetypal ground rule regarding missed sessions is to hold the patient responsible for the fee for that hour and to not see another patient during that time period—this is the most frame-securing response available. In addition, when patients announce a pending absence, the therapist should be in his or her office awaiting the patient for the full length of time allotted for the session. This is necessary because a therapist who has established the secured frame archetypal fee-related ground rule should expect to be paid for the time and thus should be in his or her office accordingly. Furthermore, in a very small percentage of cases, the patient will show up for the session despite having informed the therapist to the contrary.

Having offered some initial considerations regarding the handling of fees, I turn now to the most notable fee issues that arise in managed care settings. Their most telling effects are usually mediated outside of the awareness of the patient and of most therapists, but they are profound and deeply affecting nonetheless. They deserve our detailed attention.

AN IMBALANCE IN COST AND SACRIFICE

There is a striking contrast in managed care therapies between the cost to, and financial sacrifice made by, patients as compared to the financial sacrifices and penalties paid by their therapists. This imbalance causes therapists to suffer far more than their patients who, in a sense, benefit rather than suffer monetarily. This inequality tends to adversely affect both parties to these treatment situations, therapists more than their clients. Patients tend to experience a lesser commitment to treatment than they would in a secured-frame, private psychotherapy for which they would pay a full and substantial fee. They also tend to experience guilt, almost all of it deep unconsciously, because of the low overall payment made to their therapists and the small size of their contribution to that fee. This guilt is compounded when a patient misses a session and either is not charged a fee or only pays his or her co-pay so the therapist loses some or all of the fee for that hour. Because the attendant guilt is experienced deep unconsciously, it tends to unwittingly prompt patients to engage in self-damaging, self-punitive decisions and behaviors. In an otherwise well run psychotherapy, pressured by this kind of deep unconscious guilt, some patients will make the unwise decision to prematurely terminate their treatment. The main ameliorative in this kind of situation lies with therapists' alertness to incidents that bring up this inequality and their exploitation and properly processing and interpreting the patient's responsive encoded narratives. The use of trigger decoding is quite helpful in lessening the adverse effects of these frame deviations on managed care patients.

As for managed care therapists, these fee inequities are likely to evoke resentment toward, and envy of, their patients and anger toward the insurers who, often for unjustified self-serving reasons, set unduly low fees for treatment. These conscious and unconscious feelings and attitudes can prompt therapists to intervene in ways that are harmful to their patients—and themselves. The best way to deal with this problem is to engage in self-processing efforts when these issues are activated. This can enable a therapist to access his or her own deep unconscious experience of the situation and determine how it ties to his or her early traumas and the death anxieties that these incidents have engendered. Work of this kind can enable therapists to maintain their emotional equilibrium in the face of these destabilizing pressures and help them to avoid uncalled-for verbal attacks on, and other abuses of, their patients.

As a helpful perspective on this problem, it is well for a therapist to appreciate that he or she has willingly and knowingly signed a contract with a managed care insurer that includes a particularly low fee structure. This decision usually is based on turning to accepting managed care patients as a way of initiating or supporting one's practice especially in situations in which a therapist is having notable difficulties in getting referrals of private psychotherapy patients. Therapists join managed care networks in the expectation that the increase in the number of patients whom they see and work with will, despite the relatively low fee scales, provide them with the total income that they need in order to earn a reasonable livelihood. Smaller fees from many patients and their insurers substitute for higher fees from the fewer patients seen in private practice. Fee-wise, doing managed care psychotherapy is a trade off that means having an adequate income but also accepting a measure of financial abuse from both patients and insurers.

Nevertheless, even though therapists enter this arrangement knowingly and of their own free will, most of them feel that they are being exploited and predated by the insurers—and in most cases, this is an accurate perception. There are many valid, consciously recognized reasons for this belief—for example, the inequality of the fees paid by one insurance company compared to another; the large salaries paid to the insurer's executives; the huge profits earned by some managed care insurers; the negative publicity about insurance company executives who have engaged in dishonest or shady financial dealings; the tendency of insurance companies to reduce the fees paid to providers without prior notice; and the failure of most insurers to try to help providers keep up with the increases in the cost of living that take place each year. There also are unconscious reasons, most of them based on therapists' own deep unconscious archetypal insights into and wish for the ideal frame, which would not have insurers in the picture at all, and if they are present as a necessity, would have them pay therapists their accustomed fees.

Therapists' primitive deep unconscious experiences of these predatory frame violations join up with their conscious resentments about being underpaid and they tend to prompt therapists to make countertransference-based interventions, verbal and frame-deviant, that unwittingly convey their resentment against both their managed care patients and their insurers; through displacement, these inappropriate behaviors and verbal assaults may also be directed against figures in therapists' daily lives. If not adequately self-processed and neutralized, these deep unconscious experiences of being exploited also tend to cause disillusionment in therapists about their therapeutic work. In many cases, a self-defeating decision to stop seeing managed care patients is made and the therapist then suffers financially as well as from deep unconscious guilt and its dire consequences for abandoning individuals in need of and deserving their help. Even therapists who continue to see managed care patients suffer from a measure of this kind of guilt because they are seeing their patients under less than ideal conditions; here too both conscious and unconscious perspectives on the necessity to do so lessens the therapist's degree of self-condemnation.

All in all, we see already that doing managed care psychotherapy is an especially difficult undertaking. It is beset with a minefield of problems.

Some insurers contribute to these fee-related problems in yet another way by paying psychiatrists a larger fee for psychotherapy-medication management sessions than they do for psychotherapy sessions alone. This inequity encourages medical providers to prescribe psychotropic drugs to their patients and some psychiatrists allow the fee reward to bias their thinking as to whether or not to do so. As a result, the decision to medicate may be a genuinely valid one, but it also may have been inappropriately affected by the lure of a higher fee per session. In some instances, medical providers have responded to this arrangement by falsely billing insurers for the higher fee even though they have not prescribed medication for the patient. This is an inexcusably destructive and blatantly dishonest practice that has no place in psychotherapy, managed care or otherwise.

THE DEMEANING EFFECTS OF THE LOW FEE

A common consequence of the low fee paid to managed care therapists is the feeling of degradation experienced both consciously and unconsciously by both patients and therapists. Patients may believe that they are being seen by a less than competent psychotherapist and therapists often feel that they are right, that if they had greater skills, they would be seeing private patients exclusively. These degrading viewpoints need to be ferreted out and resolved consciously and deep unconsciously. Clinical experience indicates, however, that this issue seldom arises manifestly in the material from patients and that the problem is compounded because patients are consciously inclined to overlook and deny signs of actual incompetency in their therapists. The ultimate correctives in these situations are the therapist's offer to the patient of a truly sound, unconsciously validated therapeutic experience and his or her ability to hear and trigger decode themes in patients' narratives that have a bearing on this issue.

Maintaining one's integrity and self-esteem as a managed care psychotherapist requires continual self-monitoring, work that is carried out in the face of countless obstacles and personal resistances. The lack of stature inherent to the therapist's position with managed care patients is aggravated by a similar lack of status and influence in fashioning their contracts with insurers and in dealing with the practical problems that arise with them from time to time—abrupt treatment practices are not uncommon. Some therapists throw up their hands and stop offering managed care therapy, much as some patients terminate their managed care treatment because they feel demeaned by their insurers and, when in poor hands, by their healers as well.

DISHONEST FEE PRACTICES

I turn now to one of the most serious issues connected with fees, that of fraudulent practices. Based on the many medication consultations that I have carried out with patients who have seen other psychiatrists for medication management or who are seeing non-medical therapists for psychotherapy, indications are that many therapists consciously believe that the impoverished fees that they are being paid by insurers gives them license to violate their managed care contracts in a variety of dishonest—criminal, if you will—self-serving ways. The often do so in the face of blatant denials of the outright destructiveness of these practices for themselves and their patients. Indeed, in most instances, both the dishonesty and the adverse effects on all concerned are denied and obliterated by both parties to therapy. Nevertheless, blindness to the truth of a situation does not eliminate those truths; instead it tends to increase the severity of the consequences of these illegal interventions.

Interventions of this kind are reflections of therapists' greed, dishonesty, lack of integrity, professional moral and ethical failings, and all and all, the failure to meet their responsibilities to their patients—and themselves. The damage caused to all concerned in this manner is enormous. Most of these criminal acts go undetected by the insurer even though they contribute to higher insurance costs for beneficiaries and lower fees for providers—and thereby victimize everyone concerned with managed care treatment. A criminal therapist cannot serve as a healthy role model for his or her patients, nor can he or she produce an honest therapeutic cure.

At times, the proposal to falsely bill an insurer is suggested by patients, especially those who miss sessions either with advance notice (for which no fee is due to the therapist) or without such notice (in which case, the patient is responsible for the full fee and is asking the therapist to illegally shift most or all of that responsibility to the insurer). These invitations for therapeutic misalliances through shared corruption have wide-ranging negative effects on the course of a psychotherapy and they also damage the lives of both parties to the therapy. Dishonest frame and boundary violations soon become illicit ways of coping with trauma and anxiety for both patient and therapist. There is no constructive, curative value to these kinds of behaviors by therapists even when the rare patient reacts paradoxically to this corruption and temporarily seems to function better in response to his or her therapist's ill deeds. In effect, this would be a '"cure through nefarious comparison," but it almost never brings lasting peace to a patient (Langs 1985). For their part, dishonest therapists suffer a great deal from deep unconscious guilt and predator death anxiety and without insight as to why, do much harm to themselves, professionally and in their private lives.

On the whole, patients tend to consciously ignore or sanction their therapists' deceptions and only rarely do they raise manifestly expressed objections or report such incidents to their insurers. Their misguided, self-destructive collusion with their therapists tends to be unconsciously motivated and driven by a multitude of factors, among them the mandated deviant managed care frame that unconsciously motivates patients to ask for or accept additional deviations, some of them openly dishonest. In addition, these acts create the death-defying delusion or illusion that by cheating and defying the archetypal ground rules regarding the therapist's fees, the patient—and therapist—thereby are capable of cheating and defying death as the sequence to life. Both existential and predatory death anxieties may be momentarily alleviated in this way, but the negative effects of these frame violations ultimately undo these ill-gotten gains.

In many cases, under the influence of their own predator death anxieties, patients propose or accept these dishonest frame violations as a way of being punished for the harm they have done to others in the past. A more contemporaneous reason patients participate in these illicit deals with their therapists lies with their experience of deep unconscious—or more rarely, conscious—guilt over the low fee paid to the therapist. This guilt is aggravated when a patient misses a session with advance notice and does not pay the lost fee to the therapist. Along different lines, a patient's experience of the therapist's dishonesty also may support the patient's effort to sanction and excuse his or her own dishonest behaviors and immoral acts. This is a form of unconscious sanction to the effect that if the therapist behaves immorally it is all right for the patient to behave immorally as well.

These conscious and unconscious pressures and needs prompt patients to collude with their therapists against insurers, thereby creating misalliances that harm everyone involved in the deceit. No form of therapy is well served by misalliances of this kind because ultimately, both patient and therapist will suffer badly. Above all, no therapist has the right to put a patient in the position of shared criminality. To do so exploits the patient's self-destructive and other pathological needs and extends his or her emotional suffering in ways that can be refractory to treatment.

The low managed care fee paid to therapists often serves as the bad soil from which a variety of dishonest deviations spring forth. Some therapists charge for non-existent sessions in order to increase their income, while others see managed care patients for sessions of short duration but charge the insurer the fee for full sessions. In addition, some therapists will violate their contract with an insurer by charging the patient a surtax—an extra fee in addition to the patient's co-pay and the fee paid by the insurance company. Many therapists inform their managed care patients in the consultation session that this arrangement is the sole basis on which they will work with them, thereby initiating a psychotherapeutic tragedy in which all of the players suffer badly. The unconscious dread of death and unconscious experiences of death anxiety in both patients and therapists are the driving forces behind these corruptions. The outcome may be a premature termination of the therapy by the patient or an inappropriate clinging to the therapy and therapist based on the corrupt ties between them. However, as is the case with all partnerships in crime, the mistrust that these practices engender in both parties toward each other severely compromises the therapeutic alliance and on this basis, the damage done to all concerned is compounded.

In the name of human decency and honor, and in light of the enormous responsibilities inherent to being a psychotherapist, therapists simply must put an end to these practices; they have no place in the world of psychotherapy—or anywhere else for that matter.

CLANDESTINE ARRANGEMENTS

Still another kind of contract-violating deviation takes shape as secret arrangements between the two parties to therapy. I have already alluded to one such arrangement in which patients agree to pay their managed care therapists a supplementary fee for each session. Consciously, patients may do so because they mistakenly believe that this deviant-frame pact transforms the therapy into a seemingly advantageous quasi-private treatment situation. They also may be afraid that the therapist will be angered and dismiss them from treatment if they refuse to go along with this proposal. These side-contracts are illegal and dishonest, and the deep unconscious minds of both patients and therapists see the situation for what it is. As we would expect, efforts to deal maladaptively with unresolved and unexplored death-related traumas and death anxieties, and deep unconscious needs for punishment, play a notable role in this kind of proposal and compliance. While their encoded imagery cries out against the harm being done to them and their therapists through these practices, these patients almost never realize consciously that they have agreed to an illegal contract as the basis for their treatment experience, nor do they appreciate that they will suffer twice over—once as the victim of the therapist's deviant act and then as the victim of their own guilt-evoking need to conspire this way with their therapists.

An equally misguided deviation, which deceptively seems to benefit the patient but causes all manner of harm, arises when patients request that their therapists forgive their co-payment for one or more sessions—often, for the entire course of treatment—requests that are made on the basis of the conscious belief that they cannot afford the small fee involved. But here too hidden, guilt-based unconscious needs to undermine the therapy and to create self-damaging experiences play a significant role. Nevertheless, some therapists, fearful of losing these patients (and many patients will shop around until they find a therapist who agrees to this arrangement), will comply with this suggestion. They do so because they see it as a way of building up their patient load and as an opportunity to attract frame-violating referrals from these patients as well.

All in all, forgiving a patient's co-payment is a harmful violation of the therapist's contract with the insurer and an unwitting betrayal of the patient. Indeed, overindulging a patient in this way is much like being a mother who can't say "no" to her child—it supports the very psychopathology that the therapist is supposed to be helping the patient to resolve. Not surprisingly, the over-gratifying psychotherapist is consciously over-idealized, but deep unconsciously perceived as predating—seducing and harming—the patient. This too is a practice that has no place in sound psychotherapy.

In principle, whenever a therapist has a frame-related choice, electing to invoke or sustain a secured ground rule is to be preferred to modifying it. Adhering to this basic tenet can spare both patients and therapists much harm and grief. And given that the conscious minds of all humans, patients and therapists alike, tend to be easily corrupted and inclined toward modifying rather than securing ground rules, therapists who make this principle part of their therapeutic ethical code are armed in a way that can help them to stand fast against their patients' pressures to deviate and their own inevitable urges to act in unnecessarily frame modifying ways as well. A deep commitment to secured frames does, however, require more than an intellectual commitment from the therapist in that he or she also needs to have worked through and mastered his or her death-related traumas and the death anxieties that they have evoked. Much the same applies to the patient, which is why such work is a critical part of the treatment experience.

OTHER THIRD-PARTY SPONSORS

Another common fee problem arises when someone other than the patient is the primary insured, as when a child or adolescent is covered by a parent's policy or a spouse or significant other is covered by his or her partner's insurance. These arrangements brings a frame-modifying intruder into the managed care treatment situation. While patients tend consciously to accept these situations, their encoded messages indicate that their deep unconscious experience is once more at variance with their conscious thinking—at bottom, they feel that their therapy belongs to the insured rather than themselves. When an incident related to this frame issue arises and the patient's material permits, these unconscious perceptions need to be worked over in the therapy in order to minimize their adverse effects; failing that, premature termination is a not an uncommon outcome under these circumstances. On rare occasions, insightful processing of this trigger—which, for the patient, is constituted as the therapist's frame-related intervention of agreeing to see the patient under these conditions—reveals ample deep unconscious perceptions of disloyalty on the therapist's part. Trigger decoded interpretations along these lines may then prompt the patient to find the means of either obtaining his or her own insurance coverage or of paying for the therapy on his or her own—a frame-securing decision that is, despite therapists' best interpretive efforts, seldom made.

"Middlemen"

In many locales, insurers contract with organizations created by therapists and others—I call them "middlemen"—whose main functions are to receive referrals from the insurers and requests for therapy from beneficiaries, and to pass patients on to providers who have contracted with them to see these patients. These middlemen usually do the billing for the therapist and collect the fees from the insurer. The fees paid by the patient and insurer are shared by the middlemen and their providers, almost always on the basis of terms that are unfavorable to the therapist. Some middlemen serve mainly to complete and forward to insurers the forms needed for a provider to collect his or her fees; they usually receive and record payments from insurers and sometimes from patients as well.

In these cases, there is a strong frame-modifying third-party presence that may seriously interfere with the necessary safety and commitment to treatment needed from both patient and therapist to ensure a sound therapy experience. Patients are likely to be erratic in their attendance to sessions and therapists may be inclined to do shoddy work with these patients. When fee questions arise, providers tend to refer their patients to the middleman, thereby sanctioning a host of added deviations regarding the privacy and confidentiality of the therapy—deviations that are inimical to effective treatment.

Therapists who consent to these arrangements tend to feel demeaned because they have not received these referral themselves and because the fees that they earn are lower than the usual managed care fees. These self-perceptions tend to be shared by their patients as well, consciously and especially deep unconsciously. The many harmful effects of these arrangements call for a reassessment by both providers and insurers as to whether viable psychotherapy can be carried out under these conditions. A therapist's lack of awareness of the unconsciously mediated adverse consequences of these arrangements only makes matters worse than otherwise.

At the very least, therapists need to obtain narrative material from their patients when issues related to these arrangements arise so they can provide their patients with the trigger decoded insights needed to minimize their adverse effects. When possible, it is advisable to consider rectifying this frame deviation as both unnecessary and harmful to all concerned—except of course, the middleman. In principle, the fewer the number of unneeded frame modifications and the fewer the number of intruders, the more healing the therapeutic frame.

A frequently asked question is whether therapists should accept credit card payments from their patients. In principle, it is quite clear that doing so introduces another unnecessary third party into the therapy and that it blatantly violates the privacy and confidentiality of the treatment situation. It also is a device that distances the therapist from the patient—one that speaks for a therapist's primary interest in the fee rather than the patient.

Along related lines, a therapist should express a preference for payment by check rather than cash, even when small amounts of money are involved. As noted earlier, checks should be deposited with the words "for deposit only" in the endorsement because this assures the patient that the payment has been put into the therapist's bank account rather than cashed in a manner that leaves open the possibility that the therapist has not reported the payment as income. Given what we know about human nature and the often compromised ethical position of conscious minds, therapists are well advised to unobtrusively and without comment to their patients make use of this safeguard, thereby offering them implicit assurances of their honesty in dealing with financial matters.

MISSED SESSIONS

Another major set of already noted fee issues accrues to the problem of handling sessions missed by patients and the related question of dealing with sessions missed by their therapists. The contract offered to providers by most insurers explicitly states that the insurer is not responsible for missed sessions—that is, that they are committed to pay only for services rendered. Furthermore, some contracts also state that a patient is not to be charged for missed sessions when he or she has given their therapist 24- or 48-hour advance notice.

Therapists can suffer a substantial loss of income because of these mandated ground rules, which disregard the fact that most psychotherapists work by appointment and cannot—let alone, should not in the interest of securing the framework of therapy—readily fill hours that are freed up by patients a few days before their scheduled sessions. These mandated ground rules are, then, exploitative of therapists and they also support irresponsibility on the part of their patients, some of whom repetitively cancel sessions in advance for frivolous reasons. Such behaviors greatly undermine a patient's therapeutic experience and its outcome.

Dynamically, because they are being exploitative of their therapists, patients who cancel hours in this manner suffer from the self-punitive syndrome that is fashioned by deep unconscious guilt and predator death anxiety, while their victims—their therapists—experience predatory death anxiety and its sequelae. The exploitation of this ground rule by patients also tends to evoke considerable conscious resentment in the therapists who are victimized in this manner. These feelings may lead to inappropriately angry interventions and dishonest frame-related acts on their part, often in the form of falsely rationalized decisions to dishonestly bill the insurer for these missed hours. This practice, which may involve conscious permission from the patient, is, as noted, deeply destructive to both parties to treatment. The deep unconscious guilt it evokes in both parties to therapy wreaks havoc with the treatment experience and by extension, the personal lives of both parties to such therapy.

Because insurers allow for advance cancellations of sessions by patients, the proper handling of pre-announced missed sessions is fraught with conflicting choices for managed care therapists. Ideally, the therapist should override this deviant managed care ground rule by establishing the patient's responsibility for the full fee for missed sessions regardless of the cause or of advance notification of the therapist. Some therapists establish the rule that patients should pay their co-pay for all missed sessions, but this is a compromise that has both frame modifying and frame securing features—recall that the ideal ground rule is that the patient is responsible for the full fee for missed sessions.

Most insurers will accept therapists' modifications of this highly questionable ground rule, although Medicare and Medicaid stand fast on their position that without exception, patients are not to pay a fee, however small, for canceled sessions. Nevertheless, for misguided reasons of their own, many therapists have decided to not invoke this frame-securing tenet lest it cause problems with both the patient and the insurer. On the other hand, when a therapist does, in the consultation session, invoke the ground rule of patient-responsibility for all missed sessions, a surprisingly large number of patients fail to register it consciously—an obliteration that comes to the fore when a missed session actually arises.

Patients vary greatly in their response to the invocation of the archetypal ground rule of full responsibility for all scheduled sessions. Based on repetitive encoded images from their deep unconscious mind, which consistently supports this policy, some patients will accept their accountability for the full fee, while others will, despite their own deep unconscious advocacy for the ground rule, oppose its use. Their response depends in part on the extent to which they consciously have come to appreciate the importance and healing qualities of a maximally secured managed care frame. The intensity of their past death-related traumas is another factor, as is the extent of their dread of secured frame moments and the existential death anxieties that they evoke. Patients with severe forms of this anxiety may react by abruptly terminating their therapy without knowing the underlying reasons for this precipitous act. As for patients who continue in treatment and pay the therapist's full fee for a missed hour, the most frequent short-term result is the emergence of long-repressed, early-life death-related traumas in a form that permits their working through and resolution; symptom relief then follows. We see again that the experience of a secured frame moment does indeed open the door to deeply effective therapeutic work.

Another caveat involves the earlier mentioned secured-frame principle that therapists should not be paid twice for a given therapy hour. Consider, for example, a scheduled session that is canceled by a patient well in advance. The therapist may elect to not see another patient during that time and forgo the absent patient's fee, possibly including the co-pay, in order to hold the frame secured. But the therapist may instead decide to see another patient during the canceled hour. If so, the choices available to the therapist are quite unsavory: On one hand, he or she may choose to not tell the patient of the consultation because it involves a third party, while on the other, the therapist may decide to tell the patient of this decision even though it is a frame-deviant self-revelation that also introduces a third party into the first patient's treatment experience. All in all, it is best to keep the frame secured by not seeing another patient during the missed hour and in addition, if another choice is made, to not collect more than one fee for that time, be it from the patient or the insurer.

When it comes to dishonest practices by therapists, they have much to learn from the highly moral and ethical deep unconscious minds of their patients—and from their own deep unconscious wisdom and morality through self-processing efforts as well.

To quote Sir Walter Scott:

"Oh, what a tangled web we weave,
When first we practice to deceive."

Missed Consultation Sessions

A difficult problem arises when a patient misses his or her first appointment with a therapist, with or without advance notice. If advance notice is given to the therapist that the patient is canceling the session, little can be done regarding the fee for the missed hour even though the patient should, for reasons that include his or her own emotional well being, be responsible for payment of the fee. A different but related set of issues arise when a potential patient simply fails to appear for the consultation appointment. If he or she does not make further contact with the therapist, it is appropriate for the therapist to mail the patient a bill for the missed session, charging the patient the fee that is paid by the insurance company. Given the deviant-frame conditions of managed care therapy and the absence of personal contact in these cases, the therapist who has not established the relevant ground rule at the time of the initial telephone call will find it all but certain that the patient will not pay the fee. Even if the therapist has chosen to state the ground rule when the patient calls to make the first appointment—a practice that is frame-securing but may create conscious mistrust in the prospective patient—the patient still is not likely to pay the fee for the missed hour. Largely because many if not most managed care patients call several therapists when seeking a single consultation, this kind of delinquency is a not uncommon phenomenon in this treatment modality.

With patients who cancel their first appointment in advance of the hour but then ask the therapist to reschedule the consultation, if the patient is then seen, the encoded themes will call for payment for the missed initial appointment. But here too many patients consciously object to paying the fee even though, as we would expect, their encoded imagery speaks for the need for the patient to accept that responsibility. Therapists should not manifestly challenge this position, but should keep in mind that if at all possible this frame break needs to be rectified. In some cases, the patient eventually will come back to this problem and encode a self-imposed demand that the patient pay the delinquent fee. Trigger decoding this narrative imagery will usually prompt the patient to take care of the matter. In any case, early on, the therapist should make clear that the patient is responsible for all future scheduled sessions for which the therapist is available—that is, for any subsequent canceled hours. Failure to secure the frame in this way opens the door to further damaging frame violations and creates a context that is likely to lead to a poor therapeutic experience and outcome.

PATIENTS' FEE RESPONSIBILITIES

In addressing some words of deep unconscious wisdom to managed care patients, I would stress the need for them to develop an understanding of the seemingly forbidding subjects that are central to adaptive thinking.

The call for ethical and moral integrity applies to managed care patients as much as to their therapists. Patients should, in time, largely through their therapists' unconsciously validated efforts at frame-related, trigger-decoded interpretations and rectifications, come to appreciate the far-reaching effects of their therapists' handling of rules, frames, and boundaries. They also need to learn to mistrust their own natural propensities in this regard, especially their inclinations to accept or ask for unnecessary frame alterations. In time they also need to appreciate that frame modifications are counter-productive and ultimately harmful, while in contrast, invoking or holding fast to secured ground rules is very much in their best interests. In principle: As goes the frame, so goes the therapy.

Much therapeutic and educational work needs to be carried out by therapists in order to help their patients become "frame wise" and to gain their support in counteracting the ways in which the mandated frame violations of managed care psychotherapy presents them with inappropriate and damaging models of frame management and adaptation. This understanding, which relies greatly on their therapists' own appreciation of the role, function, and extensive consequences of the nature and management of the ground rules of therapy, can help patients to grasp the healing powers of frame-securing interventions. It also will help them to avoid contentious requests of their therapists for frame deviations like the forgiveness of their co-pay, changes in the time of their sessions, make-up sessions, and a host of other harmful alterations in the securable ground rules of managed care treatment.

In principle, patients are well advised to not knowingly propose changes in the ground rules of their therapy or in their contract with their insurers, nor should they participate with their therapists in unneeded frame alterations. There is, however, one exception to this constraint and it involves patients who can afford private psychotherapy. Accepting the change from managed care to private treatment is, as a rule, a highly favorable move for a patient and should be undertaken whenever possible.

Despite this fact, patients seldom directly (consciously) ask for this change, but those patients who can afford to do so will ask for it deep unconsciously. This encoded request seldom appears early in the course of a managed care treatment experience. More often it emerges in disguised fashion as a corrective expressed in patients' dreams and stories in response to an active, frame-deviant trigger that arises well into the treatment experience. The interpretation of this deep unconscious recommendation and wish, along with efforts to fulfill it, will have a positive effect on the patient even though it also will activate his or her secured-frame, existential death anxieties. This latter development often threatens the frame-change and may jeopardize the therapy. Making the change depends, then, on the therapist's ability to recognize the harbingers of this anxiety and on his or her using the patient's narrative images to interpret its deep unconscious sources. This is perhaps the most rewarding frame change possible in a managed care therapy and ideally it is carried out entirely at the behest of the patient's deep unconscious, encoded messages. It often requires considerable therapeutic skill and work, however, before a patient consciously accepts his or her own sound, deep unconscious advice and acts accordingly.

In practice, patients who make the change to private treatment often eventually reveal painful traumas that they have unwittingly and without realizing kept secret in the managed care part of their therapy. This is an example of how modified frames support the unconscious suppression of material connected with the trauma-related, deep unconscious sources of patients' symptoms and how securing the frame typically undoes these obliterating defenses. It is all but impossible for a patient or therapist to know that this kind of repression and denial is operating under the somewhat unsafe, modified conditions of managed treatment. Only a frame- securing moment can bring this to the fore, almost always through encoded rather than manifest images. Because the trauma involved is intimately linked to the patient's emotional dysfunctions, the therapeutic work that can be accomplished in a newly secured frame is considerable.

Implicit to this discussion is the need for patients—and their therapists—to understand the role that death and death anxieties play in their emotional problems, its psychotherapy, and their daily lives. Death is to this day a forbidden, avoided subject, but as I have emphasized it is the fundamental source of both emotional maladaptations and highly creative adaptations. Patients need to appreciate the core issues that arise as they try to cope with problems related to trauma, illness, and death itself.

ANOTHER CLINICAL VIGNETTE

Recently, a male supervisee presented a psychotherapy case to me that was relevant to this discussion. The patient was a married, female business executive who was being seen in managed care treatment. Some months into her therapy, themes in which the absence of safeguards, such as those against falling off the roof of a building, began to emerge. The imagery was triggered by a treatment report that the therapist had to complete for the insurer and by a recent substantial raise in pay that the patient had received. The material led to insights into how unsafe she felt in the therapy and into how private therapy would give her the boundaries and protective safeguards she wished for—and never had as a child. She then dreamt of a blind child, an image that brought to mind a newspaper story of a man who was blinded by a chemical accident but lacked the money to restore his vision. The imagery led to the realization that the patient would be able to see and understand her emotional traumas and their consequences only if she accepted private treatment and its cost—in the managed care therapy, she was blind to her deepest issues.

Despite this imagery, the patient considered terminating her therapy rather than shifting to private treatment, but with more help from her deep unconscious mind, she decided to make the change. A few months into the private sessions, she reported a dream in which she is kidnapped by a teenager and held hostage for a ransom. Associations led to a newspaper story in which a friend of a young girl's older brother had been playing with a gun and had accidentally shot and killed the girl. The patient also recalled a movie in which a brother trapped his sister in his bedroom and fondled her sexually. With the help of the therapist's trigger-decoded interventions, the patient dimly recalled being assaulted sexually as a teenager by her much older brother. She had doubts that it was an actual memory but further encoded imagery pointed to the reality of the assault. The patient was able to link this trauma to one of the reasons she had sought treatment, namely, her inclination to pick fights with her husband and her inability to enjoy sexual intercourse with him.

After a long silence, the patient came back to the story of the girl who was accidentally murdered. She now recalled that when she was quite young there was a lot of talk in her neighborhood about a baby who had accidentally been run over and killed by her mother. The hour ended before this last imagery could be further worked over.

This material suggests that as long as third parties were privy to the patient's therapy, she felt endangered and that her life was threatened. Based on this deep unconscious experience, she did not manifestly reveal or encode one of the major traumas in her early life. With the shift to private treatment, which brought her the safety she needed and also evoked secured-frame entrapment anxieties, she was able to encode and deal with the early trauma the secured frame had activated—namely, her brother's sexual assault. This repressed incident had a significant connection to her emotional symptoms.

The initial association to the accidental killing of a young girl evidently was a condensed image in that it alluded first to the patient's brother's sexual assault on her, and second to another, probably earlier death-related trauma that was further encoded in the story of the mother who accidentally killed her baby. In subsequent sessions, the patient's encoded imagery centered on other themes of parents harming children and stories about abortions. While the patient did not consciously recover a memory of her mother having had an abortion, the therapist used this material to reconstruct such an event—and he obtained encoded validation for his efforts.

The secured frame was the trigger that facilitated the patient's direct recall of one early death-related trauma and the encoded recall of another such event. It can be seen, then, that the conditions of treatment have a profound effect on what patients remember consciously and encode unconsciously. As noted, the extent of these effects and the hidden secrets that are shut off by the frame-modified aspects of managed care therapy cannot be known without a shift to private treatment. Indications are that major traumas that are pertinent to the etiology of a patient's emotional maladaptations may not materialize because of the dangers posed by the mandated managed care frame deviations. The degree to which this is the rule and the depths of their effects are matters in need of further clinical study.

A final note of caution for managed care patients: It is well to pause to think through any decision they make to prematurely terminate their therapy. In the hands of a frame-modifying or otherwise harmful therapist, this may be a highly adaptive, wise decision. But as we have seen, this decision alternatively may be a reaction to an effective therapist's frame securing and trigger-decoded/interpretive efforts and thus be highly maladaptive and unwise. With the exception of blatantly inappropriate and assaultive or seductive therapists, with whom termination is a sound choice, the denial-plagued, unperceptive, poorly informed conscious mind has no way of differentiating adaptive from maladaptive decisions of this kind. In contrast, the wisdom system of the deep unconscious mind knows precisely the reasons for the wish to leave treatment and thus, turning to narratives and trigger decoding holds the answer to this dilemma. If their therapist does not make use of these techniques, patients are well advised to try it on their own.

To shift now to a few related words to therapists, it is critical that they not react manifestly in favor of or against their patients' seemingly premature thoughts of terminating their treatment. Instead, they should encourage the expression of narratives in order to give the patient's deep unconscious mind an opportunity to encode its wisdom and point to the triggers and anxieties that are provoking this decision; as a kind of full service system, the imagery from the deep unconscious system also will allude to the consequences this decision will have for the patient—and therapist. If the flight is indeed unconsciously motivated by the activation in the therapy of one or another form of death anxiety, the deep unconscious mind will allude to this problem and strongly advise the patient to stay in treatment. On the other hand, if the decision is well advised, the encoded themes will so indicate. By and large, patients—and all humans—consistently speak the truth only when they speak indirectly through encoded narratives.

PATIENTS' REACTIONS TO THERAPISTS' DISHONESTIES

Situations in which therapists intervene in grossly dishonest ways present a host of uncalled-for difficulties for their patients. It is not uncommon for one or both parties to therapy to consciously ignore or obliterate the deviant enactment by the therapist. This is the case because deep unconscious wisdom and morality have little effect on conscious thinking and thus do not affect and lead to sensible conscious responses to therapists' dishonest interventions. In addition, patients' predator death anxieties and unconscious needs for punishment will motivate them to accept an illegal frame break by the therapist because they will suffer from the harm it does to them—the conscious effects of the deep unconscious system of morality and ethics are considerable. Then again, for its part, the deep unconscious mind is extremely sensitive to this type of intervention and will strongly object to being made into an unwitting accomplice of, and partner in crime with, the deceitful perpetrators of these immoral deeds.

In this regard, some principles of conduct for patients can be articulated. Patients faced with a dishonest therapist should bring up the problem manifestly and directly with the therapist. In addition, they should examine the themes in their dreams and associations to their dreams for their unconscious view of the situation—doing so with or without the help of the beleaguered therapist. Denial is not a factor in deep unconscious perceptions and the patient's encoded imagery will involve brutally frank images pertaining to the dishonesty involved and the harm and mistrust being caused to the patient—that is, the ways in which these interventions are destroying the therapeutic process, experience, and outcome.

With therapists who fail to desist in such behaviors, the patient should consider leaving treatment and think about notifying the insurer of the problem. This situation often involves issues of criminality and malpractice that are the province of criminal investigators and state boards of licensing; each case must be dealt with incisively but individually. All in all, then, the handling of this most serious matter must be carefully thought through consciously by the patient, who should do so with help from his or her own deep unconscious wisdom system and system of morality and ethics. In some cases, this working through needs to be carried out with the aid of a new therapist who, it goes without saying, must have more integrity than the therapist in question. The therapist's being able to trigger decode patients' narratives also is of great help in these matters.

It is to be stressed, however, that while patients' conscious objections to their therapists' dishonesties and other frame modifications are likely to be valid—these tend to be blatantly deviant interventions—these conscious assessments need to be confirmed through the patient's encoded imagery. These situations are very different from those in which patients manifestly complain about their therapists' adherence to a secured ground rule or criticize their interpretations—only the deep unconscious mind knows for sure how valid these criticisms are. The latter type of objection may arise on the basis of patients' unresolved existential death anxieties and thus are inappropriately defensive and in error; they will not be supported by patients' encoded thematic images.

Finally, it is clear that even when a patient participates in a therapist's fraudulent act, the therapist himself or herself must bear the greater burden for what has been done and for the negative consequences for both parties to therapy that emerge as a result. More broadly, therapists must understand that they have the primary responsibility for managing the ground rules of managed care therapy even when a patient is the prime mover for a frame-deviation. Although both parties to treatment have responsibilities for the therapeutic outcome, therapists are much more accountable than their patients for the success or failure of the treatment experience.

PATIENTS' REQUESTS FOR FEE CHANGES

As noted earlier, some managed care patients ask their therapists to forgive their portion of the fee. This is, of course, a frame-violating request that ill serves the patient and will not be supported by his or her own deep unconscious mind and the encoded imagery it emits. For their part, when such requests arise, therapists who do not work adaptively should not respond directly to these requests and should try to explore the direct and encoded material that ensues. Adaptive psychotherapists can rely on their patients' encoded directives to tell them to not comply to such a request. It is noteworthy, however, to realize that this kind of request is quite rare in their work because they are inclined to secure as many ground rules as possible for their managed care efforts. To turn around a maxim I've often cited, secured frames beget secured frames—they tend to preclude both requests from patients to modify the ground rules and frame-violating behaviors on their part.

To be clear, the deep unconscious mind realizes that the truly impoverished patient—and they are quite rare—is better served by terminating treatment until he or she can pay the co-pay rather than eliminating this element of financial responsibility for the patient. This frame-securing intervention is a far more therapeutic alternative to therapists agreeing to make exceptions of this kind. Indeed, this type of frame deviation is highly toxic for both parties to therapy; showing the patient that his or her unconscious mind is opposed to his or her conscious appeal is the best way to manage this type of incident.

The therapist who goes along with this request is to some extent bribing the patient to remain in treatment. He or she also is making the patient an exception to the managed care contract and ground rules of the therapy, a move that increases the patient's inappropriate sense of entitlement and inclination to deal with trauma and stress by destructively modifying frames in both psychotherapy and everyday life. Much harm has been wrought through these false act of kindness by therapists, who, by agreeing to this request, also demean themselves. Deep unconscious guilt is activated in both parties to such an arrangement, which is thereby another consciously overlooked way of damaging a psychotherapy experience.

Narrative-based explorations indicate that unresolved death anxieties motivate this type of frame modification. Indeed, for this reason patients propose an almost endless array of self-destructive, frame-altering collusions with their therapists. For their part, therapists should, in principle, trigger decode and interpret the unconscious basis for these demands rather than accede to them. As a rule, a previous, therapist-evoked frame deviation is the intervention that activates this kind of request by patients. Therapists must therefore be mindful of ways in which their own frame violations have unconsciously encouraged and sanctioned their patients' wishes to act in similar fashion. A therapist's ability to hold the frame secured when asked by his or her patients to deviate, to rectify a frame violation that has contributed to the suggestion, and to interpret the deep unconscious meanings involved in this kind of interlude converts a potentially damaging situation into one that is distinctly healing.

THE ABSENCE OF A CO-PAY FROM THE PATIENT

An especially difficult and somewhat misguided mandated ground rule for some forms of managed care psychotherapy—for example, those that are sponsored by Medicaid—states that patients are not responsible for any part of the fee paid to the therapist. Clinical experience indicates that this ground rule creates an especially unstable and treacherous framework for the therapy, one that causes much harm to all concerned. Under these conditions, both patients and therapists tend to engage in unneeded frame modifications, many of them exploitative of the other party to therapy. Unannounced absences and abrupt terminations by patients, and inexcusable dishonest fee practices by therapists, are quite common under these conditions.

Under these circumstances, therapists best serve their patients by agreeing initially to work with them as mandated and look for opportunities to secure this ground rule as well as other unneeded frame deviations when possible. Despite these hazards, which slow the progress of treatment, a successful long-term outcome of treatment is feasible though arduous. A five- or ten-dollar co-pay would go a long way toward partially securing this frame breach and would offer some much-needed structure and responsibility to both parties to the therapy—changes that could well lead to faster and deeper cures than seen otherwise. Trigger-decoded interpretations of the patient's deep unconscious experience of this fee arrangement help to stabilize these situations, but these patients are loathe to listen to their own deep unconscious objections—and they are abundantly conveyed—to this self-serving yet harmful fee arrangement.

Ironically, any effort made by a therapist to secure the frame by establishing a small co-pay for each session or by holding the patient responsible for the full fee for unannounced absences tend to be barred by the managed care contract for these patients. Because their unconscious death anxieties are mollified but not resolved by this arrangement, they tend, when the issue does come up, to either consciously insist on sustaining the no-pay frame deviation or abruptly terminate their therapy rather than tolerate its securement; indeed, they can easily find other therapists who will not question this arrangement. Therapists who realize the damage that is being done in this way face considerable resistances in trying to deal with these situations in ways that help their patients to heal their emotional wounds, but the effort should be made nonetheless.

UNPAID FEES

Another difficult fee-related problem arises with patients who owe their therapists money. Common causes lie with patients' forgetting to bring their copayments, interludes when the patient's deductible is in play, or situations in which an insurer turns down a bill submitted by the therapist because the patient is not covered for the sessions in question—that is, a patient is seen by a therapist on the basis of tentative approval by his or her insurer only to discover that the coverage is not in place or has elapsed. In some cases the insurer rules that the patient is suffering from a pre-existing condition and therefore must wait months before the insurance becomes active. Under these circumstances, many patients leave treatment rather than agreeing to pay the fee themselves, while others do so before their responsibility for the fee becomes apparent. The therapist is entitled to the fees for these sessions and should bill the patient accordingly, but he or she must do so on the basis of the insurer's fee schedule. Nevertheless, under these circumstances, many patients will fail to pay their final bill, thereby creating a basis for their own unconsciously orchestrated guilt-related suffering and presenting a real and often daunting problem for the therapist to handle.

The options open to therapists in these circumstances range from resigning themselves to the loss of income to hiring a collection service to collect the unpaid fee. Direct appeals to the delinquent patient by mail or telephone should come first, but they seldom are effective. Thus, it usually comes down to biting the bullet and taking the loss or bringing a third party into the therapy in order to rectify the patient's frame-deviant, predatory behavior. Invoking this frame-deviant option is justified because of the patient's own frame-deviant behavior in not paying what he or she owes the therapist. Collection agencies charge therapists fees for their services. Because of this, in the consultation session, some therapists ask their patients to sign an agreement that states that they will accept full responsibility to pay for legal and collections fees if they fail to honor their commitment to pay the therapist's rightful charges. In many cases, however, this agreement violates state laws and is illegal; its use therefore is ill-advised.

As can be seen, there is no ideal solution to the non-payment of fees by beneficiaries. Those therapists who accept this situation with resignation are unwittingly supporting their patients' frame-violating dishonesty and lack of ethics and morality. But on the other hand, they also are holding the therapy frame secured by not involving a third party in the treatment—albeit it in a way that allows the patient to exploit them. Therapists who elect to turn to collection agencies when it is an entirely legal option are challenging rather than sanctioning the patient's frame-deviant dishonesty, but in order to do so, they are bringing outsiders into the treatment. Therapists have no control over the practices of bill collectors, who may badly expose and harass the delinquent patient. Yet the patient's frame violation and predation of the therapist has brought such behaviors down on him or her. That said, therapists also must look to their own frame-management practices to identify any frame-deviant triggers that have contributed to their patients' delinquency. While this does not justify the patient's behavior, it does offer a perspective on the problem that can affect the therapist's ultimate decision as to how to most fairly deal with it.

Given that issues are raised by each of the choices available to therapists in these situations, they should be aware of the pros and cons of each possibility, including the conscious and deep unconscious ramifications for themselves and their patients. In making a final decision, therapists who have contributed to the situation by breaking the frame should be mindful of their role in the patient's behavior—and take in a lesson well learned on this basis. In these situations, responsibility for the patient's non-payment must be shared by both parties to the therapy, a fact that should not, however, necessarily prevent a therapist from collecting the fees that are his or her due—it should, however, give pause for thought.

THE TIMING OF A THERAPIST'S COLLECTION OF FEES

A few last words on therapists' handling of the fees for therapy. As I have said and shall emphasize in the following chapter, fee management should be the responsibility of the therapist alone; no third parties should be involved. Problems arise, however, in regard to the ideal ground rule of accepting payment for sessions at the beginning of each new month for the previous month's sessions. Therapists readily make this kind of arrangement for private patients, but there are reasons they tend to be hesitant to do so with patients seen under managed care auspices.

The heart of the problem lies with the finding that, unconsciously buttressed by the basically deviant frame of the therapy in which the insurer pays most of the therapist's fee and the patient pays a rather low co-pay, many patients consciously feel entitled to see their therapist without accepting any financial responsibility for treatment. In a few words, they expect a free ride. Among the consequences of this false sense of entitlement are patients' failures to pay unpaid co-pays following the termination of treatment. It follows from this that a therapist who arranges for patients to pay their co-pay at the beginning of each month for the previous month's sessions risks non-payment when the patient leaves treatment. Given that this happens quite often, it seems unwise for a therapist to adopt this archetypal tenet; instead, he or she should be paid the co-pay at the end of each session, though never in advance of a session. My personal experience with this small alteration in the ideal ground rule is that it does not evoke negative deep unconscious reactions and seldom becomes a significant trigger for patients' deep unconscious experiences of the therapist and therapy.

A CLOSING COMMENT

All in all, it can be seen that the archetypal ground rules regarding therapists' entitlement to a fair and appropriate fee for their services and their patients' responsibility to pay that fee themselves raise a host of frame-related issues in managed care psychotherapies. Each of these issues involves questions that pertain to the best way to secure as much of the frame as is possible. Each also presents both parties to therapy with a minefield of dangers that could adversely affect the therapeutic process, its outcome, and the emotional state of both patient and therapist. Each also is strongly influenced by deep unconsciously experienced forms of death anxiety, which wreak havoc with conscious efforts to properly manage fees in managed care therapies. Accessing the patient's—and a therapist's own—death-related deep unconscious wisdom and morality as connected with fee-related dilemmas takes therapists a long way toward finding the best solution to these often daunting problems.

It is often said that the truths of nature are in the details. While the conscious mind tends to overlook many details, the deep unconscious mind is not so inclined. This means that in dealing with fee issues, therapists are well advised to listen to the smallest bit of encoded theme because it may hold the clue to the resolution of a fee-related problem. That said, I turn now to the other ground rules of managed care psychotherapy so we can look at the problems and issues that they too raise.

Chapter Seven

Other Ground Rules of Notable Influence

I turn now to the other archetypal ground rules that have significant effects on the managed care psychotherapy experience. A detailed look at these rules is called for because collectively, they have a broad and telling impact on the psychotherapy experience and crucially affect both patient and therapist. In addition, each individual ground rule, when it is secured or modified, tends to have major effects on the treatment experience as well; their handling by the therapist often holds the key to the success or failure of the treatment. I begin with the two ground rules that, after therapists' fee, loom largest in the managed care scene—privacy and confidentiality.

PRIVACY AND CONFIDENTIALITY

Privacy and confidentiality, which generally go hand-in-hand, are two of the most important pillars on which the archetypal psychotherapy frame is built. Some years ago, a survey of emotionally ill patients who had decided to not seek the psychotherapy they needed revealed that about 15 percent of respondents avoided therapy because of concerns about confidentiality, while another 10 percent said they stayed away because their health insurance did not pay enough for mental health treatment or counseling.

These findings suggest that in addition to patients' deep unconscious concerns about the adverse effects of the inevitable departures from the archetypal frame in managed care psychotherapies, there are influential conscious worries as well. Nevertheless, when seen in consultation, managed care patients tend to consciously deny that they are concerned about the privacy and confidentiality of their treatment. They invoke this denial even though the violation of these rules, be they small or large, is part of the basic framework under which they will be seen. It is noteworthy that this denial is belied by the finding by adaptive therapists that in their consultation and early therapy sessions, most patients will encode unconscious concerns, anxieties, and reservations about violations of these two components of the archetypal frame. Indeed, their violation accounts for much of the uncertainty, instability, and limitations—whatever they may be—of managed care psychotherapy and for its predatory qualities as well.

The extended version of the archetypal ground rules in respect to privacy and confidentiality may be stated as follows:

A psychotherapy experience should be conducted with total privacy, that is, without third-party intrusion in any manner. Neither the patient nor the therapist should directly or indirectly introduce another person, agency, or institution into the treatment situation. Thus, they should not discuss any aspect of the therapy with an outsider nor expose anything about the treatment experience through the written or spoken word. There should be no note-taking or recording of the transactions of the therapeutic interaction by either party to treatment. Furthermore, the psychotherapy should be conducted in a manner that guarantees the total confidentiality of the entire treatment experience. Outsiders are to be excluded from gaining information about, entry into, or access in any way to the therapeutic transactions during the therapy as well as before or after it is initiated and ends. Psychotherapy should be an evanescent experience without the creation of temporary or permanent records of any kind.

This statement describes a therapeutic ideal that is universally sought and consistently validated by deep unconscious minds even as the conscious minds of both patients and therapists adopt varying views and attitudes about the importance and maintenance of these two ground rules. Nevertheless, these tenets are vital aspects of the framework of psychotherapy in that they serve to protect both parties to treatment from unnecessary exposure to and harm from others, and assures them the security and safety essential to insightful emotional healing. For patients, these rules are strongly related to matters of trust, the reliability and devotion of the therapist to the patient's therapeutic needs, and the protection needed for the revelation of horrendous traumas at the hands of loved ones as well as the patient's own darkest secrets. Insight therapy is grounded in the working through of the death anxieties evoked by the reactivation and re-experience of these traumas and their psychologically disfiguring effects on the patient. The recall or reawakening of these experiences, both consciously and unconsciously, poses dangers for both patient and therapist—dangers that are mollified by adherence to these two archetypal ground rules of treatment.

Despite these adaptive findings, the fact is that these two essential, ideal ground rules are at a variance with some state and federal laws, which, because they are based on advisories from ill-informed conscious-system psychotherapists, run counter to the optimal therapeutic environment and ground rules needed for a sound psychotherapy experience. Motivated by the conscious proclivity for modified frames, the standard approach of organizations to the framework of psychotherapy tends to be strongly frame deviant and the negative consequences of frame violations are greatly underestimated or ignored entirely. Proper redress is called for.

As already indicated, both total confidentiality and total privacy inevitably are modified in managed care psychotherapies. It is difficult to envision a way in which the situation could be otherwise. Even when the patient pays the full fee to the therapist and then receives some part of the fee from the insurer, the patient must reveal information about the therapy—at the very least a date of service and almost always, a diagnosis. The goal, then, must be to find ways to minimize these modifications of privacy and confidentiality so as to reduce their effects on the patient, therapist, and treatment process. Adherence to the principles of adaptive psychotherapy can facilitate the identification and working through of the most disruptive and disturbing aspects of these deviations. Such work often will turn a harmful situation into a compelling, insightful therapeutic interlude.

Achieving these goals requires overcoming a variety of obstacles. For many reasons, some of them entirely unfounded and treacherous, adherence to total privacy and confidentiality is quite rare in any form of psychotherapy in use today. Therapists of all persuasions seldom think through or appreciate the implications and consequences of seeing the parents of children or adolescents, the spouses of married patients, or the relatives or intimate friends of other patients whom they are seeing in treatment. Similarly, they are not inclined to educate their referral sources to have the patient rather than a relative or the referring professional himself or herself make the call for the patient's first appointment with the therapist. In addition, referral sources need to be taught to avoid calling the therapist to provide information about the referred patient—therapists should get all of their information from patients themselves. If the referring party does call, the therapist should see to it that the call is brief and as uninformative as possible. That said, exceptions to these rules of conduct may arise with patients who are in a psychotic state or who are homicidal or suicidal. As with all frame-related issues, the basic rule of frames holds true here: Always secure as much of a ground rule as reasonably possible.

In principle, then, managed care psychotherapists should keep intrusions of third parties and modifications in confidentiality to an irreducible minimum. Aside from the insurer, to whom a bill must be sent and who, for some patients, requires information to authorize future therapy sessions, a therapist should not be in contact with outside parties for any reason short of a dire emergency. This means, for example, that unless a patient is suicidal, homicidal, or in a psychotic crisis, therapists should not accept or return calls from third parties. Privacy is the best policy.

SOME FREQUENT ISSUES

Third-Party Psychiatrists

A frequent source of third-party issues lies with situations in which a patient is being seen by a non-medical psychotherapist for psychotherapy and by a psychiatrist for medication management. It is not uncommon for the referring therapist to call the psychiatrist to tell him or her about the reasons for the medication referral and to request a return call after the patient has been seen. But as is the case with so many aspects of psychotherapy, this approach, which is unnecessarily frame-violating, is based entirely on conscious-system thinking without consideration for deep unconscious archetypes and preferences. The practice of having the patient sign a release and give written permission for the discussion to take place does not modify the frame-deviant qualities of the situation, nor does it lessen the unconscious impact of the contact on all three parties to the frame violation. That said, if a therapist and psychiatrist do engage in this ill-advised policy, written permission from the patient must precede their doing so. In addition, after the discussion takes place, both parties have the responsibility to inform the patient as to what transpired.

In addition to the very real and consequential objections of the deep unconscious mind to this practice, there are conscious reasons to be skeptical of its usefulness. For one, these frame violations have two parties speaking about the patient in his or her absence, a situation that is likely to evoke mistrust and conspiracy-theory, paranoid responses. Even when one or both parties to this situation tell the patient what was said, the patient is likely to mistrust the report (and it is likely to be significantly incomplete or even distorted) and to feel exploited and endangered. The patient also is likely to wonder whose interests are being most served, those of the treating individuals or his or her own. Worries about collusion, kickbacks, and the secret aspects of the nature of the relationship between the two therapists are to be expected—and if they do not emerge consciously, as often is the case, they will materialize in the patient's encoded narrative imagery. Indeed, as noted, the deep unconscious mind strongly objects to these conversations and experiences them as predatory rather than helpful. Such practices need to be reconsidered and discarded as running counter to the archetypal needs of patients—and their therapists—in respect to the two ground rules we are exploring at the moment.

Other Third Parties

The principle of keeping to the optimal frame holds true in situations in which patients consciously make requests of their therapists to bring other kinds of third parties into the treatment situation, directly or by telephone or email. This request may—or should—include the offer by the patient to sign a release that permits the therapist to modify one or both of the ground rules under consideration.

In these cases, there are two basic ways the therapist can deal with the situation. The first and less effective approach is to explore the patient's conscious reasons for the request and if the patient does not withdraw it, agree to release information only if it is deemed to be absolutely necessary—and kept to an absolute minimum. The second approach entails the use of adaptive principles of technique such as eliciting dream material and other sources of narrative images in order to gain access to the patient's encoded, deep unconscious perceptions of the meanings and consequences of the therapist's compliance with such a request. These narratives will include encoded advisories as to how the situation should best be handled—and they always favor keeping the frame as secured as possible. With utmost regularity, then, this effort will enable the therapist to identify the triggering event that has unconsciously evoked the patient's frame-modifying request—most often it involves a frame modification by the therapist. On this basis, the therapist is in a position to interpret the patient's deep unconscious insight into the sources of the request and his or her objections to the very frame violation for which the patient has petitioned.

There are, of course, situations in which the patient's request that the therapist release information to a third party appears to be quite necessary. Patients who are suffering from disabling psychological problems and are in need of a disability report, others whose insurance coverage requires reports from the therapist, and those who have been mandated to enter therapy because of some kind of criminal or socially objectionable act or behavior and for whom the court requires a report on the treatment—these are the kinds of patients for whom the therapist has no choice but to release the necessary information and thereby modify the patient's privacy and confidentiality.

As for therapeutic principles for dealing with these situations, the therapist must be certain that the information to be released is vital to the interests of the patient and the continuation of his or her therapy. In addition, the therapist can comply with these requests only with the patient's written permission that he or she may do so. The information to be forwarded should be shown to the patient before it is transmitted to the third party and modified at the patient's request only if there are legitimate reasons to do so. There must be no attempt to manipulate the information transmitted in a misguided effort to present a picture that is unduly and inaccurately favorable to the patient. Complete honesty is essential. Finally, the therapist should be prepared to treat this release of information to a third party as a frame-deviant trigger that the patient may or may not work over consciously, but certainly will deal with deep unconsciously.

Along different lines, some patients seek therapy because of a court mandate or because they are involved in litigation and expect the therapist to send a report on the therapy when called for. In principle, a therapy whose framework requires from the outset that the privacy and confidentiality of treatment will be violated for reasons of this kind is almost certain to be manipulative on the part of the patient and likely to have as its primary goal the success of the patient's legal cause. The therapist who accepts a patient for therapy under these conditions is agreeing to a frame-deviant contract that first and foremost will have him or her representing and exposing the patient in court rather than healing his or her emotional ills. The patient's deep unconscious view of the therapist is likely to be one of corruptibility, untrustworthiness, and a demeaned tool of the patient. Mistrust of the therapist also is likely, as will be a tendency, both consciously and unconsciously, for the patient to conceal unflattering and disturbing material and to favor presentations that advance his or her cause. For these reasons, it is best for both the patient and therapist for the therapist to not accept the patient into therapy with this proviso and to offer an alternative plan, namely, that they do therapy without the expectation of the release of information and that the patient see another therapist for the evaluation related to the litigation in which the patient is involved—if such is needed. Effective psychotherapy cannot be conducted within a framework in which non-therapeutic goals are primary and questionable violations of confidentiality and privacy are inherent to the treatment process.

Other Therapists

Another largely unnecessary but frequently enacted modification of privacy and confidentiality involves requests for information about patients who have terminated their managed care psychotherapy with one therapist and have gone on to see another therapist. In many instances, the second therapist will call or write to the previous therapist asking for details about the first therapy. The patient's written permission must, of course, be obtained, but providing such information is a frame violation and is, with few if any exceptions, a useless gesture that is harmful to all concerned. There is no way that third-party information of this kind can help the new therapist in treating the patient because the therapist must learn about the patient's therapeutic needs and emotional problems through his or her immediate interactions with the patient—that is, from personal experience. This is all the more the case because, short of a disaster in the life of the patient, the essence of what a patient communicates, especially on the deep unconscious level of expression, is always triggered by the interventions made by the current therapist. It follows then that the information that a prior therapist could provide to a current therapist is stale and of no viable use for the new therapist or for the patient. In all instances, more harm than good is done in these cases.

SOME OVERALL PERSPECTIVES ON PRIVACY AND CONFIDENTIALITY

Taking an overview, we can see that the deep unconscious mind is rightfully and uniformly opposed to violations of these two privacy-centered ground rules of psychotherapy. This position applies to both their mandated and arbitrary violations; responsive themes of undue exposure and betrayal are abundant when departures from these tenets occur. On the whole, however, the deep unconscious wisdom system has an especially jaundiced view when these ground rules are unnecessarily violated by a therapist—and it often is accompanied by a modification in his or her anonymity. At such times, the remarkably perceptive deep unconscious mind, as reflected in its narrative expressions, will detect clues that these decisions have been evoked by a recent death-related trauma that has activated of some form of unresolved death anxiety in the therapist—and almost always this assessment is right on the mark. *The deep unconscious mind knows that abrupt unneeded frame violations almost always are triggered by a current death-related trauma*. It follows, then, that therapists who suffer from a death-related issue personally are well advised to be on the lookout for inclinations to unnecessarily modify the archetypal frame—and they should refrain from doing so. Self-exploration through self-processing is called for in these situations—trigger decoded insights are invaluable in helping therapists avoid traumatizing their patients and themselves under such trying circumstances.

Patients in managed care psychotherapy make unconscious allowances for mandated frame violations, but nevertheless the deep unconscious mind is relentlessly ideal in its position on the ground rules of therapy and the ethical position of the psychotherapist. Detoxification of the harm done by deviations in these two areas can come about only by working through the patient's deep unconscious responses to these frame modifications, that is, by detecting and utilizing the models of rectification—that is, the frame-securing correctives—offered by the patient.

In psychotherapy sessions, every fresh violation of a patient's right to privacy and confidentiality evokes narratives that convey deep unconscious perceptions of the inappropriate exposure, betrayal, and harm that is being done to the patient—and therapist as well. These interventions create a climate of mistrust that may be felt consciously, but seldom mentioned directly by the patient. Under such conditions, the psychotherapy often is severely compromised: Patients are unconsciously motivated to withhold embarrassing and otherwise disturbing personal material and to obliterate traumatic historical events in which loved ones and others have played seductive and destructive roles. They also tend to avoid manifestly criticizing therapists who act frivolously in violating these tenets, even as they deep unconsciously rightfully see the therapist in a starkly negative light. Mistrustful paranoid-like responses are common, as are disturbances in the therapeutic alliance; the justified fear of further exposure by the therapist plays a major role in these reactions. Here too offending therapists will experience deep unconscious guilt and suffer accordingly—especially if the frame deviation is gratuitous and unneeded. And unresolved death anxieties unconsciously hover over these incidents in ways that can be detected solely through the use of trigger decoding.

THE INSURER AS THE THIRD PARTY TO THERAPY

Insurance carriers generally ask for a relatively small and reasonable amount of information in respect to the initial sessions of a managed care psychotherapy. In the main, all that is required is the patient's identifying data, diagnosis, type and date of services, and the therapist's contracted fee. Insurers also require that therapists keep adequate general notes and in some cases, therapists also are also allowed to write and file additional process notes to which no one other than the therapist has access. Much of this is a matter of the state and federal laws that define these requirements and needs, in principle, to be followed. Patients do have the right, however, to ask their therapist to release this material to third parties for various justifiable reasons, a matter that has been discussed above.

Turning now to another frequent problem in managed care psychotherapy, some insurers require that providers who wish to continue their patient's psychotherapy beyond the number of sessions that are authorized initially must complete an outpatient treatment plan that requires the release of specific information about the patient and the therapy. Insurers' policies vary considerably in this regard, ranging from giving the therapist the freedom to continue the treatment without authorization to asking the therapist to provide very detailed information about the patient and the therapeutic transactions. In general, the more frequently a patient is seen regularly each week, the greater the amount of information that is sought from the therapist by the insurer.

It is, of course, advisable and necessary for therapists to comply with a given insurer's policies as stated in their contract, but the information released should be as general as possible and must be shared with the patient before sending it to the insurer; this is a way of reducing the extent of the patient's paranoid and mistrustful reactions to these submissions. The therapist's goal should be to prevent the undue exposure of the patient and to limit what is revealed to a basic minimum. Insurers need to be educated about the consequences of frame modifications so they can weigh the pros of a maximally secured frame against the cons of their sponsoring a psychotherapy that may not be viable. This understanding would provide them with a better perspective on the amount of information that they actually need regarding a psychotherapy experience in order to authorize its continuation. In many cases, this is far less than currently requested.

That said, if therapists were to behave, work, and theorize in ways that encourage a greater trust of insurers, the latter might well be inclined to give up the request for clinical material as the basis for authorizing further treatment and rely entirely on the judgment of their contracted therapists in this regard. As I discovered while serving on a review panel for one of the main mental health insurers, present policies by insurers are, in part, the result of their being faced with compromised or dishonest billing practices and grossly incompetent therapeutic work carried out by their psychotherapists. Clearly, every act of dishonesty by a patient or therapist harms not only themselves and their insurers, but also the entire universe of patients and therapists. There is much truth in and consequence to the old cliché: "Honesty is the best policy."

On a related matter, some insurers require that a mental health provider be in contact with and send information to a patient's primary care physician. This is another conscious-system-wrought, highly damaging, frame-modifying policy that arises in the context of complete ignorance of frame-related archetypes. Even on the manifest level, such communications, which would need the patient's prior written approval based in his or her examining the material to be transmitted, is another frame deviation that is bound to make patients mistrustful of, and feel harmed by, their therapists. If at all possible, this kind of third-party contact should be avoided by the therapist—it is of little if any value.

SOME BASIC THERAPEUTIC PRINCIPLES

In principle, in their consultation sessions, therapists should inform their patients as to the nature of the information that they are obliged to release to an insurer. As noted, in most cases, all that is required at first is the patient's diagnosis and dates of services. The patient also should be informed that beyond this information, the treatment will (and should) be both private and confidential, and that nothing personal will be recorded or conveyed to others by the therapist—nor should anything be recorded or spoken about to others by the patient. Subsequently, when additional information is required by the insurer in order to approve the continuation of the therapy—or the patient of absolute necessity asks that information be released to another third party—the nature of this released information also should be imparted to the patient. As I have indicated, patients seldom will address the resultant frame issues consciously, but they will, of course, react deep unconsciously and encode their unconscious experiences in their dreams and stories. This narrative material, which encodes and deals with actual consequences of the frame modification, can then be interpreted to the patient in light of their triggers—in these cases, they are constituted as the therapist's frame-violating revelations about the patient.

This kind of work is highly therapeutic because of its honesty, integrity, and ethical qualities—all the more so if frame-securing rectification is feasible and carried out. These efforts reflect an appreciation of, and genuine empathic attunement with, the patient's intensely affecting deep unconscious experiences. In addition, the therapist's acceptance and implicit validation of the patient's deep unconscious perceptions of the meanings of a given deviation constitutes an implicit acknowledgment of the measure of harm done by his or her action. There is, however, no need for the therapist to adopt a consciously confessional stance; working with and accepting the patient's imagery as inherently valid unconscious perceptions of his or her intervention is all that a therapist need do to establish damage control in these trying situations.

When insurers keep their requests for patient information to a minimum, patients can be seen in managed care psychotherapy under the best possible conditions in respect to privacy and confidentiality. At the very least, because personal details are (or should be) omitted, they can be assured of the confidentiality of their personal revelations to their therapists. It must be stressed again, however, that while these reassurances may be accepted consciously, they are never fully trusted deep unconsciously. As a result, themes of third-party intruders who expose and damage the patient, and of mistrust and persecution, are not uncommon in managed care therapies. Indeed, the managed care psychotherapy frame is inherently paranoid-making and when patients develop that kind of thinking, it is incumbent on their therapists to recognize the triggers that account for the emergence of these symptoms; therapists' immediate or recent frame-modifying interventions make a very real contributions to their development. As always, the best way to turn these traumatic experiences into moments of insight and healing is by interpreting and working through patients' encoded deep unconscious responses to the frame violations at issue. Failure to do so can create serious risks that include therapeutic stalemates and failures, displaced paranoid reactions to individuals in the patient's outside life, and unconsciously driven paranoid reactions to the therapist himself or herself, which may lead to premature terminations of the therapy. There are many serious risks for both patients and therapists in therapists' failing to properly interpret the deep unconscious ramifications of these frame violations.

THIRD-PARTY INTRUDERS ON BEHALF OF THE THERAPIST

Another very common breach of privacy and confidentiality arises when providers engage secretaries to be involved in such matters as making appointments, greeting patients, and doing their billing. In similar fashion, many therapists hire professional services to do their billing and handle inquiries into fee issues. Such practices are not uncommon, especially among medicating psychiatrists and very busy managed care psychotherapists.

Providers who see a large number of patients under managed care conditions are hard-pressed to do their own billing and they often engage someone else for this task and for taking care of their voluminous paperwork. This frame violation, which manifestly modifies the ground rules pertaining to fees (the archetypal ground rule calls for the therapist to do his or her own billing) as well as privacy and confidentiality is justified by conscious-system psychotherapists as a practical necessity. Nevertheless, the intention to do so should be measured against the fact that it does involve a series of potentially harmful frame violations. There also are manifest drawbacks to these arrangements such as patients being aware of this third-party presence and, as a result, becoming mistrustful of the therapist, and the likelihood that an employee will make errors for which the therapist, who often is quite unaware of these mistakes, must bear responsibility. Secretaries and billing services who interact directly with patients also may make untoward comments and behave in ways that are manifestly harmful to patients. Here too damage is done, but the therapist usually is unaware of it and yet is ultimately and responsible for it having happened—the deep unconscious mind rightfully holds the therapist entirely responsible for these incidents. It is well, then, for therapists to keep in mind that ideally, their practices should be theirs alone and that thoughts of bringing in third parties should be scrutinized carefully, explored through self-processing efforts that include trigger decoding, and avoided if at all possible.

Therapists who nonetheless bring third parties into their offices and engage them in billing their patients should take precautions to avoid the all too frequent abuse of patients that takes place under these circumstances. One of the more difficult questions to answer is whether the therapist should inform the patient in the consultation session—or later if need be—of the third-party arrangements that he or she has made. When a secretary or assistant makes the therapist's appointments and when a billing service bills the patient and collects the fees from the patient and insurer, their presence is self-evident and the patient should be forewarned. As I have stressed, patients will seldom react to or bring up this practice consciously—and if they do mention it they tend to accept its use or simply raise practical questions when they arise. Nevertheless, the frame deviation will evoke deep unconscious reactions that have a great deal of silent but negative influence on both parties to the therapy. Therapists need to engage in narrative-based explorations with their patients and in private self-processing on their own as ways to minimizing the harm done by these arrangements. Doing so can, once more, turn these situations into sources of deep insight and healing for the patient—and, at times, for the therapist as well. In principle, interpretation supported by rectification—that is, the therapist's decision to forgo the services of the intruding third party—is the ideal approach to this frame deviation.

In some of these frame-deviant arrangements, the therapist collects the patient's co-pay and the billing service deals only with insurers. Under these conditions, the therapist may be justified in not revealing this intrusion to the patient because the information is the private business of the provider. There are, however, several precautions that should be taken in this connection. For one, there should be no direct contact between the secretary or billing service personnel and the patient. For another, if the patient becomes aware of the third party, his or her presence should be acknowledged by the therapist and then processed through the patient's manifest and encoded material. In any case, if a fee issue arises, it is the therapist's responsibility to explore and resolve it with the patient—as noted, the billing service should not have direct contact with the patient. Much the same applies to any issue that comes up between the billing service or secretary and an insurer—the therapist should be the person to negotiate the problem.

In addition to taking measures that would render the third-party intruder as invisible as possible to the patient, the therapist should be on the alert for encoded themes that touch on this frame deviation. This alertness is needed because the patient may well have either consciously become aware of the third party and immediately repressed and obliterated this awareness or may have experienced the presence of the intruder entirely unconsciously without the least amount of conscious awareness. Thus, therapists who bring third parties into their practices should be on the alert for themes like secret intruders, financial errors, mistrust, and the like in order to appreciate that the patient is, for good cause, reacting to this trigger deep unconsciously. Therapists must meet patients' images half way: They must listen for frame-related themes in general and when a specific frame-securing or frame-modifying intervention has been carried out, they must be on the alert for themes that bridge from encoded stories to the frame issue at hand. All the while, the therapist must take care to not lie or deceive the patient about these third-party presences—falsehoods would only aggravate an already aggravating situation.

Along different lines, therapists should make clear to their billing personnel that the information that they will be working with is confidential and should not be shared with or mentioned to anyone other than the insurer. Under these conditions, there always is the risk of leakage largely because of the human inclination to modify ground rules and frames far more than to adhere to or secure them. Here too, should a lapse occur, the therapist must bear full responsibility for the frame break. Therapists who maintain as much privacy and confidentiality as possible can serve as role models for those whom they employ; contrariwise, therapists who are careless and frame-violating unconsciously encourage and inherently sanction frame-violating behaviors in their employees.

Once a third party is brought into the billing process, it is imperative that the therapist not expand the use of that individual for additional frame-deviant purposes. The most likely extension of tasks for busy managed care practitioners involves having the secretary answer the telephone and make appointments for the provider. Such practices bring an imposing third party into the therapeutic relationship and he or she becomes yet another obstacle to the patient's need to have, as much as possible, an intimate and safe one-to-one relationship with the therapist. This also is a way in which therapists quite inappropriately and unnecessarily distance themselves from their patients and deep unconsciously, patients will see the third-party presence as a reflection of their therapist's fear of being alone with them. Despite the therapist's rationalizations for this arrangement, his or her patients will unconsciously and accurately perceive indications that some form of unresolved death anxiety underlies these deviant arrangements. Deep unconscious mistrust of, and feelings of being predated by, the therapist are among patients' likely responses to these intrusions. These reactions need to be detected in patients' narrative material and interpreted accordingly; rectification of the deviation is an important additional measure.

Another kind of third-party intruder recruited by managed care—and private—psychotherapists comes up when they take vacations or a leave of absence from their practice. These covering therapists or psychiatrists are, of course, third parties for the original therapist's patients and they therefore entail serious breaches of privacy and confidentiality. Here too patients tend to consciously accept these intruders unless they do something grossly untoward. Nevertheless, as we would expect, this practice is decried deep unconsciously and as a result, it leads to the kinds of negative reactions described above.

Consciously it would seem that a therapist is between a rock and hard place in connection with this matter. On the one hand, there is an apparent need for therapists and especially medicating psychiatrists to have emergency coverage in their absence, but on the other hand, the frame violations involved may have devastating effects on the patient—and often on the absent therapist as well. On balance, the best solution to this dilemma is in keeping with the maxim that calls for the most frame-securing choice available, which is to not bring a third party into patients' treatment experiences. Even consciously, this choice seems best because short of an emergency absence, therapists can fully prepare their patients for the interludes during which they will be away from their offices, including medication coverage. Then too, should an emergency arise—and in a well-run practice, they are extremely rare—patients can turn to their primary care physicians or go to an emergency room for the care they need. In addition, years of practice have shown me that no therapist can be responsible for the way other therapists practice their trade. In addition to the leakage of information about the patient that is part of this kind of situation, invited therapists often intervene in ways that are highly damaging to patients and the patient often will repress what happened even as he or she is adversely affected, often in serious ways. The original therapist must bear responsibility for these untoward interventions and the damage caused may well be beyond repair—symptomatic regression and abrupt termination by the patient may transpire. Thus, the damage done by the frame violations that are inherent to this arrangement is usually compounded by lapses made by the invited therapist, thereby making the entire experience untenable for all concerned. There also is the added problem of the borrowed guilt that the referring therapist is likely to suffer when matters go awry. This adds up to the advice that therapists should avoid such arrangements and keep their practices to their own. Conducting a managed care practice is difficult enough without adding on the burdens created by a colleague.

SOME ADDITIONAL THERAPEUTIC PRINCIPLES

In terms of technique it is to be emphasized that therapists who bring seemingly unseen third parties into their work with patients need to keep an ear open for encoded themes that indicate that the patient has been involved with or knows about the presence of the intruder—consciously or deep unconsciously. If leakage occurs, patients seldom mention it directly, but they do react deep unconsciously and encode themes of invasion, unwelcome guests, people who are afraid of being alone with madmen or madwomen, and the like. If not detected by the therapist and processed through the narrative material, these secrets can cause much harm to the patient and the therapeutic process. The therapist must be alert enough to play back the encoded themes in patients' narratives that suggest that something of this kind is in play.

The therapist should not, however, unilaterally bring up the subject of a third party directly if the patient has not already done so. This kind of intervention is a frame-violating self-revelation that entails a breach in the therapist's anonymity and it typically evokes denial-based conscious responses even when it turns out the patient did have relevant manifest information. Indeed, many patients who consciously experience an acute frame violation will subsequently repress or obliterate the entire incident to the point where they will not recall it under any circumstances—even when the patient's material enables the therapist to allude to it directly. With these patients, the therapeutic work must be done solely on the deep unconscious level of experience using the patient's narrative imagery and playing back the themes that convey the patient's obliterated perceptions. In addition, therapists will do well to monitor and process their own narrative images for expressions of their personal deep unconscious guilt for bringing a harmful third party into their practice no matter how justified the move may seem. These are delicate matters with many adverse effects that are mediated deep unconsciously. Encoded themes hold the key to their resolution.

PATIENTS' RESPONSIBILITIES REGARDING PRIVACY AND CONFIDENTIALITY

It is not generally appreciated that the ground rules pertaining to privacy and confidentiality apply not only to therapists, but also to their patients. In framing and structuring an ongoing psychotherapy experience—which should, as a rule, be carried out in the consultation session—a therapist should first indicate what he or she will, with the patient's written permission, be required to reveal to the insurer. The therapist should then indicate that the specific material from the patient's sessions will not be recorded in any manner, nor used for any secondary purpose whatsoever. He or she should then go on to advise the patient that it is in his or her best interests to also keep the therapy private and confidential, and to not record or discuss any aspect of the sessions with third parties of any kind.

Because of the intense interactional features of the therapeutic experience, if a patient violates either or both of these ground rules, the first step in dealing with its ramifications involves a search by the therapist for frame-violating behaviors of his or her own. Indeed, therapists' frame modifications tend unconsciously to be the triggers and motivators for frame violations by patients. Patients' frame deviations must be explored with this in mind and their narratives interpreted in light of the therapists' frame-deviant, triggering intervention—when such is the case, as it usually is. This therapeutic work is carried out in terms of both the patient's unconscious perceptions of the therapist's frame deviation and the patient's own need to modify the archetypal ground rules in response. Rectification through the patient's decision and pledge to desist in enacting this leakage should be based on the insights gained in this way.

In respect to the therapist's contribution to the patient's acting out, it is well to first look for recent frame modifications that fall beyond those that are mandated by the contract with the insurer and to then search for mandated frame modifications that have been activated by a recent triggering intervention by the therapist. Given the conscious human bent for frame violations, therapists' mandated releases of information about the patient to the insurer often are recruited consciously, and more often, unconsciously by patients to justify their own self-defeating, defensive, death-denying, deviant-frame needs and behaviors. Interpreting and rectifying the therapist's contribution to the patient's acting out is vital to insightfully resolving these problems.

The therapeutic interaction is a two-way exchange that takes place in a bipersonal field. With the exception of severe outside traumas, almost everything of significance that a patient says and does in therapy (and to some extent in his or her everyday life) is on the some level evoked, much of it unconsciously, by what the therapist has said and done. This is especially true of their deep unconscious experiences and thus, their encoded imagery. Thus, patients may talk about any number of different manifest subjects, thereby varying their conscious concerns, but all the while almost all of the stories they tell encode deep unconscious experiences of their therapists' interventions. In contrast, therapists are equally sensitive to traumatic events in their everyday lives and in their work with patients. In addition, almost everything a therapist says and does in the treatment situation is or should be evoked by the patient's behaviors and material. That is, therapists' communications to patients should not convey their personal narratives or in any other way encode their own deep unconscious experiences of the patient in the therapy. Instead, they should focus on the conscious job of decoding and interpreting the patient's encoded narrative imagery. This does not preclude silent moments in which a brief narrative or fleeting image comes to the therapist's mind and he quickly trigger decodes its meanings. This may well be a form of deep unconscious attunement with the deep unconscious experiences of the patient and it may, if unconsciously validated by the patient's ongoing narrative themes, prove to be a special source of insight into the deep unconscious experiences of both the patient and the therapist himself or herself. While this kind of effort should not detract the therapist from his responsibilities to listen to and deeply understand the patient, it is a valuable way for therapists to insightfully resolve the unconscious basis for their own erroneous interventions—frame-wise and otherwise.

OTHER GROUND-RULE AND ETHICAL ISSUES

Most of the other archetypal ground rules of psychotherapy can be established and sustained by managed care mental health professionals. As noted earlier, this includes a set fee; a professional locale for the therapist's office; establishing and adhering to well-defined and appropriate time constraints for the therapeutic contact; arranging and adhering to the agreed-on time and length of sessions; a reasonable vacation policy with adequate advance notice; the therapist's relative anonymity; the use of neutral interventions, however they are defined; the absence of physical contact between patient and therapist; and the therapist's basic dedication to the patient's therapeutic needs and the patient's respect for the therapist's efforts.

Here too it is well to reiterate some critical principles:

A therapist's deep unconsciously experienced image as an ethical and moral professional who is trustworthy and available to his or her patients for sound unconscious identifications may be somewhat marred at first by the mandated frame violations of managed care therapy. The therapist's integrity is expressed, then, mainly by offering unconsciously validated interpretations and establishing and sustaining the remaining ground rules of treatment—and rectifying a mandated deviant ground rule when it can be secured. These interventions not only neutralize the harmful effects of the mandated frame deviations, but also, by means of deep unconscious identifications, provide patients with effective adaptive resources. On the whole, frame-securing efforts contribute significantly to the emotional healing of the patient and to the legitimate satisfactions and mental health of their therapists as well.

With this in mind, let's look now in some detail at the basic ground rules that can be established and sustained in managed care psychotherapies.

The Fixed Frame

The "fixed frame" refers to the ground rules of psychotherapy that can be set at the outset of treatment and sustained with little or no variation as a given therapy unfolds. They include the therapists' responsibility to be present for all scheduled sessions, and his or her commitment to hold to the arranged location, day, time, and length of sessions. Also relevant is the therapist's seeing to it that contact with the patient is limited to the appointed times and locale for sessions; there are, then, no prearranged extra- or post-therapeutic contacts between the therapist and patient. With rare exceptions, the fee set by the therapist in accordance with the managed care fee schedule also should remain unchanged throughout the therapy.

These ground rules have their counterparts in the call for patients' complementary adherence to a similar set of rules—that is, to be present for all scheduled sessions; to arrive on time for sessions and accept their endings as properly announced by the therapist; to not ask for sessions to be shortened or extended; to keep to the frequency of sessions as arranged at the outset of treatment; to make no attempt to meet with the therapist outside of the time of the scheduled sessions; and to pay the therapist's fee in timely fashion. The request for an emergency session may be a legitimate, frame-modifying exception to the fixed frame, but often this proves to be a less helpful deviation than either party expects.

Adhering to these tenets provides a solid core of stability for both parties to the managed care therapeutic experience. Even so, both parties to therapy are under unconscious pressures to depart from these ideals, much of it derived from the mandated frame-deviant conditions and from their need to defend against personal, unresolved death anxieties. It is not infrequent then for one or both parties to therapy to seek or invoke unneeded frame violations that involve the tenets of the fixed frame. These frame deviations may be enacted unilaterally by the therapist, or requested of the therapist by the patient. Thus, either party to treatment may seek to change the time of a single session or may propose a make-up session for one that was missed. A therapist may begin or end a session early or late or change the patient's fee for one or more sessions. For their part, patients may arrive late for sessions or leave a session before time is up. More often than is generally seen in private practice, therapists are inclined to cancel sessions for frivolous reasons and patients unnecessarily tend to miss scheduled hours.

Technically, therapists should refrain from invoking any of these unneeded frame modifications and when patients make such proposals, they should not support or agree to the request. Instead, they should adopt an exploratory interpretive stance, seek the triggers for the request in their own interventions, and allow the patient's encoded images to facilitate insight and their sustaining the ideal frame. The already articulated principles of adaptive technique should be invoked.

An exception to these ground rules arises when a patient asks the therapist to change the time of all future sessions because he or she is making a job or other life change such as being saddled with a new, conflicting schedule of classes at school. The therapist's necessary acquiescence to these requests is frame modifying and it is therefore critical to explore the deep unconscious ramifications of this change before the therapist arranges a suitable new time for the patient's hours. This is one of those rare situations in which a frame modification is invoked in order to secure the frame in a more lasting way. Gaining deep unconscious perspectives into these frame changes and their implications tends to lessen any possible negative effects.

Special attention should be paid to the tendency of managed care therapists to be quite lax in respect to their attendance at sessions and in beginning and ending sessions at the designated times. Non-emergency cancellations of patients' sessions with or without advance notice are unjustified and anti-therapeutic. Becoming a mental health professional confers a mantle that gives the healer a powerful influence over his or her patients—an influence that may be used for harm as well as healing. This responsibility should not be taken lightly. Everything that a therapist does and says, no matter how seemingly trivial consciously, may have inordinate power deep unconsciously. There are, in truth, no trivial therapeutic interventions, especially when they involve the management of the ground rules of therapy. The unconsciously mediated adverse behavioral effects of seemingly innocuous deviant interventions by therapists are enormous. Every extended silence and verbal intervention by a therapist must be viewed as an active trigger and if possible, its effects examined through patients' encoded narrative responses. If an intervention involves modifying or securing the frame, it should be explored as a pending trigger in the session in which it arises before it is carried out by the therapist. And once it has been invoked, a second assessment of the meanings and consequences of the intervention should be made by the therapist and interpreted to the patient in light of the patient's manifest material, and even more so, with full consideration of the decoded meanings of the patient's encoded narratives and deep unconscious adaptive and evaluative responses.

THERAPISTS' RELATIVE ANONYMITY AND NEUTRALITY

Another rather common violation of the ground rules of managed care—and private—psychotherapy involves therapists' offers of non-neutral directives, personal opinions, their own idiosyncratic associations to their patients' material, and the offer of a wide variety of gratuitous personal comments and self-revelations. There are a group of dynamically oriented psychotherapists who advocate that therapists engage selectively, within ill-defined limits, in sharing aspects of their personal feelings toward their patients and in revealing aspects of their personal lives to them as well (Langs 2006). There also are many psychotherapists who engage in what they believe are justified nonneutral interventions such as aggressive confrontations of and challenging questions to their patients. Also common are therapists' use of their own thoughts and associations to their patients' material as a basis for intervening, including the often-used turn to material from earlier sessions that the patient has not alluded to in the current hour. This latter practice has been found to be extremely biased and to mainly serve the defensive needs of the therapist; these interventions seldom obtain encoded validation by the patient. Along similar lines, there also is a large group of cognitively and dynamically oriented therapists who offer their patients a wide variety of non-neutral advisories, so-called training and anti-phobic exercises, and make suggestions to their patients that come from their own thinking rather than the patients' material.

All in all, there is a host of non-neutral interventions used by all manner of therapists that are not properly recognized as severely prejudiced, frame violating, and unconsciously harmful to their patients. These efforts do not take into account patients' negative deep unconscious reactions to these widely advocated and extensively used interventions.

As for matters of definition:

Ideally, therapists' relative anonymity *entails their limiting the information that a patient obtains about themselves to inescapable revelations such as the location and furnishing of a therapist's office; his or her manner of dressing, speaking, and intervening; the kinds of interventions that he or she does and does not make; and other comparable non-deliberate self-revelations. The rule precludes intentional self-revelations and interdicts therapists' imposing their attitudes, opinions, personal advice, and the like on the patient.*

Complementing this rule is the ideal rule of neutrality, *which calls for therapists to intervene solely on the basis of their patient's material in the session at hand. This rule also precludes a therapist's offer of advisories, directives, and the like. However, it does not interdict therapists' inevitable use of their clinical and theoretical positions as background information that informs their interventions. Even so, therapists should have a sound, unconsciously mediated means of validating (or invalidating) their interventional efforts—and thereby their underlying theoretical thinking as well. Ideally, because of the defensive, denial-prone biases of the conscious mind, manifest affirmations of therapists' interventions by their patients do not serve as a reliable means of validation. Instead, confirmation of therapists' interventions should be sought in patients' responsive encoded narratives: In general, positively cast stories are affirming, while those that are negatively cast are non-validating. This is the case because patients' deep unconscious minds accurately monitor the validity of their therapists' interventions and encode their assessments in responsive dreams and narratives.*

Some Additional Issues

Departures from these two deep unconsciously sought and unconsciously validated ground rules are legion within and outside of managed care psychotherapy. Much as therapists are consciously divided on the issue of personal disclosures to their patients, the conscious minds of patients react variably to their therapists' self-revelations. Some patients find them objectionable, but most patients welcome them; in truly misguided fashion, they believe that these confessions are ways that therapists are being properly empathic and expressing their humanness. This viewpoint is not supported on the deep unconscious level of experience and it has arisen largely because, as practiced today, psychotherapy and psychoanalysis are conscious system forms of treatment that have no means of recognizing the pervasive deep unconsciously mediated harm caused by these self-exposures. The situation is further aggravated by the fact that there is no consensus as to the bounds that should constrain these self-disclosures, nor is there an appreciation for the many valid, non-deviant ways that therapists can express their empathy and concerns for, and humanity to, their patients—much of it based on tuning in on patients' deep unconscious experiences and intervening accordingly.

As we would expect, despite patients' conscious uncertainties about the effects of these self-revealing interventions, their deep unconscious minds uniformly see all departures from a therapist's relative anonymity and neutrality as frame violating, seductive, self-serving, exploitative, and damaging to all concerned. With this in mind, therapists are well advised to refrain from making such interventions and should they do so, they should trigger decode the patient's responsive narratives as valid unconscious perceptions of the offensive meanings and ramifications of these non-neutral interventions. These measures are especially necessary in managed care psychotherapies because of the instabilities and pressures toward maladaptive frame modifications caused by their mandated frame modifications.

For their part, many patients initially approach their therapies and therapists in a casual manner designed to give the relationship a social cast. They will ask the therapist about his or her personal life and professional preferences, and they often are annoyed or upset when the therapist fails to answer them—even as they are pleased deep unconsciously. Psychotherapy patients need to be educated through their treatment experiences that it is in their best interests to not request this type of frame alteration from their therapists. They should learn to be wary when therapists intervene in this manner and to accept and silently respect and appreciate therapists who do not inappropriately reveal themselves and thereby hold this part of the frame secured.

In this regard, special note should be made of patients who, in the course of their first telephone call to, or in their consultation session with, their therapist, ask pressing questions about the therapist's professional qualifications and at times, his or her personal history. Consciously, many therapists offer revelatory responses to these queries, but here too there is no conscious consensus as to where to draw the line. Some therapists will provide a limited professional history but not a personal one. This may seem like a reasonable choice, but nevertheless, it sets a frame-deviant tone to the therapy. In this context it is well to recognize that patients have no sound way of consciously evaluating a therapist's professional qualifications and there are other dangers in responding with any information at all. Thus, patients are likely to misconstrue and distort what the therapist has revealed and they also are inclined to exploit the information in order to shift the focus away from themselves onto the therapist. These self-revelations also put the patient in control of the therapy and they incite the patient to make further requests for self-revelations and frame violations by the therapist, many of them arising when the patient becomes threatened and anxious about the experiences that are emerging in the psychotherapy.

An added perspective comes from the clinical finding that even though these patients recruit the conscious argument that they are entitled to be informed consumers, with some regularity, patients who make these pressured inquiries tend to be quite fragile, mistrustful, and paranoid. They have a strong need to take charge of the therapy, tell the therapist how to do his or her job, and restrict the material they reveal to the therapist—directly and especially through the generation of encoded narrative material. They are, then, deeply threatened by dynamic forms of psychotherapy because they have a strong unconscious dread of their inner mental world and the death-related traumas around which it is organized. They tend to be very belligerent, generally inclined toward frame violations, poor narrators who tend to restrict their expression of encoded imagery, unconsciously beset with hidden death anxieties, and disinterested in obtaining symptom relief through the acquisition of deep insights. They seldom remain in a managed care therapy whose frame is as secure as possible and whose transactions they are unable to dictate.

In sum, therapists will do well to be cautious about responding directly to patients' inquiries about themselves. They should make every effort to gently adhere to non-disclosure and explore the sources of these questions in both triggering events—that is, their own frame-related interventions—and the usually severe traumatic incidents that have made these patients so wary and mistrustful of others. Thus, the best frame-securing response by the therapist to these pressures is to point out that the therapy is about the patient and not the therapist, and that the patient will learn all that he or she needs to know about the therapist by experiencing how he or she does psychotherapy.

SOME FINAL COMMENTS

We are reminded again that there are no casual communications from patients in psychotherapy and no meaningless or trivial responses by their therapists. That said, it is worth noting that these pressured challenges to therapists' anonymity that are so frequent in managed care treatment situations are another example of the extent to which handling the ground rules of managed care psychotherapy is especially difficult for therapists. In these cases the mandated frame violations invite efforts by patients to have their therapists further modify the ground rules in ways that relieve them of their underlying death anxieties. Indeed, managed care patients tend to enter treatment expecting to have a frame-deviant experience—and they do all they can to make it happen that way.

Many patients who could afford private treatment choose this treatment modality because of an unconscious investment in this feature. This adds to therapists' frame-management problems and jeopardizes sound forms of therapy because many managed care patients react adversely to frame-securing moments related to therapists' anonymity and neutrality. They ask for advisories and threaten to and often terminate if they are not forthcoming. Their dread of the world of deep unconscious memories and experiences, and the death anxieties so contained, is so enormous that if they cannot be assured that narratives will not play a role in their treatment, they are soon gone. This very common dread of deep unconscious meaning is one reason why therapists who do not work adaptively or trigger decode narrative material are so popular with patients today. The avoidance of death is the key to their appeal. And while this applies to psychotherapists seeing patients privately, it is all the more so with therapists who do managed care therapy. Such work is, as I have been trying to demonstrate, quite complex and arduous.

Chapter Eight

Some Major Concerns

I turn now to a series of problems that arise in connection with managed care treatment that I have not as yet explored in any detail. Nevertheless, they are among the more troubling concerns that arise on the basis of the mandated conditions of this treatment modality and it is critical for therapists to be as clear as possible as to the nature of these issues and the means by which they can best be handled.

ISSUES OF COMMITMENT

As might be expected, the tenuous nature of the managed care frame has an insidious influence on the commitment that the parties to therapy make to each other and to the therapeutic process. Ideally, both patient and therapist should be fully dedicated to each other in a therapeutic sense and entirely committed to the success of their joint efforts to bring emotional relief to the patient. This dedication is reflected in therapists' creating and patients' accepting a well-defined therapeutic contract and a set of ground rules that is as ideal as possible under the circumstances. Commitment also is reflected in the efforts of both patient and therapist to understand and appreciate each other's appropriate role in the treatment situation, including their respective role requirements—their nature, range, and limitations, and the frustrations and satisfactions they provide. There also needs to be an effort to grasp and understand the meanings and intentions of each other's words and actions—their sources and their consequences. This mutual devotion also is fostered when the two parties to therapy achieve genuine rather than false empathic attunement, which takes place largely on the deep unconscious level of experience.

Therapists' therapeutic commitment is expressed from the outset, beginning with their telephone contact with potential patients. During the call, the therapist should behave and communicate in a professional manner with a focus on determining the patient's need for treatment, the existence of any emergency issue, and the source of the referral. Importantly, the therapist should offer a prospective patient a consultation appointment that is not unduly delayed. If the therapist cannot see the patient within a week of the first telephone call, it is usually best to suggest that the patient make other arrangements. A referral to one colleague (but not the offer of a list of possibilities) is a viable but often risky option. In any case, if an appointment is made, the patient should be informed of the length of the session, which, in all cases including medication management, should be a full 45 or 50 minutes. Attention to details of this kind—and they include establishing and maintaining a set of ground rules that are as secured as possible—tends to assure the patient that the therapist is fully committed to his or her work with the patient.

For their part, the commitment of patients to their therapists and the therapeutic work they intend to do together also finds expression in the initial telephone call. In scheduling the first appointment, patients need to be reasonable about their time constraints and clear about their need for treatment, and they should be seeking care because of their own motivation rather than suggestions and pressures from third parties. They should keep to the appointment they have made and not ask for it to be changed; they also should be at the therapist's office at the appointed hour. From then on, an appropriate investment in therapy is expressed by their being present and on time for all scheduled sessions and by their adhering to the ground rules that have been established by the therapist in the first session.

Other factors that enhance therapeutic engagement are complete honesty and sincerity on both sides, a factor that is, however, expressed differently by patients and therapists. The former must be candid without suppressing any thought or feeling, while the latter must be sincere and honest within well-defined constraints that includes suppressing—that is, not revealing to the patient—any of their personal thoughts and feelings and anything else that is not derived from the patient's material in a given hour. There needs, then, to be a sense of a therapist's genuine integrity and uncompromised morality as well as a patient's sincere wish to constructively resolve his or her emotional difficulties. There can be no direct or implicit abuse of either member of the therapeutic dyad.

In light of these ideals, it seems clear that there are many facets of managed care psychotherapy that tend to weaken the commitments made by patients and therapists to each other and to a sound psychotherapy experience.

Every departure from the ideal frame interferes with the investment in the therapy made by both parties to therapy and thus lessens the chances of a deeply successful, constructive outcome for the patient. This finding should be appreciated by both parties to treatment. As I have been emphasizing, the conscious minds of both patients and therapists tend naturally to treat therapy in a far too casual manner and both parties are at risk of having a cavalier attitude toward their commitments to the psychotherapy situation.

Some patients approach their therapists as if they were their acquaintances or friends and they try to be casual and cool about the relationship. They try to engage in chit-chat with their therapists and to treat the contact as social rather than professional in nature. Therapists must recognize that the therapeutic relationship is different from a social relationship and that it has a particular and more stringent set of rules, frames, and boundaries. They therefore need to avoid responding in a non-professional manner to their patients' seductive overtures lest the treatment be derailed. A professional response is neither cold nor inappropriate; it is in keeping with the role requirements of the therapist and the therapeutic needs of the patient. As the deep unconscious mind knows full well, it is when a therapist responds otherwise that he or she is being cold and harmful to the patient. The therapeutic relationship is a formal one and any effort by either party to therapy to give it a more informal cast reflects a diminution of their therapeutic commitment to each other and the treatment process.

The problem of commitment is often activated and played out around patients' planned and unplanned absences from sessions. Naively and self-destructively, patients consciously tend to believe that no harm will come to them if they miss a session for frivolous reasons, but all the while their deep unconscious minds know better. It is therefore well to be aware of the serious consequences that tend to befall patients who miss sessions, especially when they fail to take responsibility for the fee for the hour—a point that is abundantly clear from the responsive encoded messages stemming from their deep unconscious minds. In an odd twist of logic, patients believe that not being charged for a missed session by their therapist shows how much the therapist cares for or about them, but their far wiser deep unconscious minds know that the opposite is the case. There is a strong and immutable link between adhering to the ground rules of therapy on the one hand, and on the other, to being committed to the therapeutic process and to one's partner in the therapy.

Patients' Commitment to Treatment

Compromises with, and impairments in, patients' commitment to their therapists and their therapies find their earliest source in the fact that most patients find their therapists through impersonal and poorly informed means such as a list of providers that says little or nothing about the qualifications of the therapist. A stronger tie to a therapist would be based on a professional recommendation in which the referring party speaks positively, albeit generally and within due limits, about the therapist's abilities and qualifications. This holds true even though the referring individual has no sound conscious means of accurately evaluating the skills of a particular psychotherapist. Still, the referring source's praise of the therapist creates an aura that enhances the patient's inclination to invest in the treatment, while the long list of providers and the absence of any encouragement tends to make the patient wary and less inclined to commit.

That said, as soon as the consultation session begins, a strong unconscious influence is activated that will most powerfully affect the extent to which the patient becomes prepared consciously to commit to treatment. By virtue of its evolved design, the patient's defense-oriented, denial-prone conscious mind is strongly inclined to favor committing to a therapist who supports these defenses. Patients who run counter to this trend are the exceptions rather than the rule. It can be said that patients are naturally inclined to commit to working with the most denial-supporting, frame-violating (and thereby harmful) therapist whose unfavorable interventions they can consciously idealize and justify. These unconscious needs tend to override the more mundane conscious considerations such as the therapist's attentiveness, empathy, evident concern, intelligence, and the like. The way in which these superficial factors are experienced is greatly affected by the unconsciously influential history of a patient's death-related traumas and the patient's ability to tolerate the generation of the narratives that give access to these incidents and their meanings and effects on the patient's emotional ills. While all of these considerations pertain to private psychotherapy, they are more troublesome in managed care treatment where the distorted frame makes it a lot more difficult to help patients generate a strong commitment to therapists who are truly deserving of their trust.

Turning to other, more practical factors that may interfere with patients' commitment to their therapists and their mode of therapy is the fact that in many locales, the therapist is but one of many practitioners available to them. The idea of significant differences in skill and qualifications among therapists seldom arises in patients' thinking. One anonymous therapist is much the same to them as another anonymous therapist, and given the conscious mind's dread of deep unconscious meaning, the relatively skillful therapist is often perceived more as a threat than a gifted healer. Patients' distancing themselves from their therapists is further reinforced by the ease with which changing managed care therapists can be accomplished and by the availability of undisciplined therapists who cater to patients' defensive needs for deviant frames and the denial of death and the death anxieties that fuel human neuroses.

Also relevant is the small size of patients' co-payments and the relatively low overall fee that a therapist receives for a managed care psychotherapy or medication management session. Yet another restrictive factor is the ease with which insurers permit patients to miss sessions with—and at times, without—advance notice and the relative lack of privacy and confidentiality of the treatment. There also are pressures from some insurers—and some patients—for the overuse of psychotropic medications, which give the effort at insight psychotherapy a diluted and relatively impersonal quality. Finally, in many cases the patient's primary commitment is far more to the insurer who subsidizes a variety of medical and emotion-related treatments than it is to the therapist. It has been said that "therapists may come and go, but insurers are for a lifetime." Indeed, the presence of the insurer and the commitment that both patients and therapists make to this third party to therapy is a major factor in the involvement issues seen in both parties to managed care psychotherapy.

There are, then, a multiplicity of external factors that play a role in the creation of barriers to the basic trust and intimacy needed for an ideal therapeutic experience. They join forces with contributions that come mainly from within patients themselves—and within their therapists as well. To clarify these inner factors, some of them already noted. Many highly traumatized patients have an aversion to sound, intimate exploratory forms of psychotherapy because of their fear of re-experiencing the death anxieties, psychological damage, helplessness, and rage that would emerge in a narrative-based reworking of the deep unconscious effects of these devastating incidents. In addition, patients who are suffering from the deep unconscious guilt and the consequences of having caused significant harm to others also dread becoming engaged in a meaningful therapy experience because on the deep unconscious level of experience they are fearful that they will punish themselves severely in response to the reactivation of these critical incidents.

Because they suffer from severe unresolved death anxieties, these patients tend to flee psychodynamic forms of therapy, especially at moments in which the obliterated issues have been triggered by some incident within or outside of treatment or when the therapist is able to secure a deviant part of the frame, however temporarily. These patients unconsciously fear commitment of any kind and as a result; they prefer to keep their distance from their therapists in part by insisting on the invocation of unneeded frame modifications. If these requests are not granted and not adequately interpreted in light of the prevailing triggers, many of these patients will terminate their treatment. Strong unconscious death anxieties lie beneath their interpersonal anxieties and these patients will keep their distance from their therapists until these anxieties are insightfully resolved—a difficult task at best.

Unmastered unconscious death anxieties are the basic psychodynamic cause of commitment failures in both psychotherapy patients and their therapists.

The practical consequences of patients' relatively diminished commitment to therapy include a greater incidence of canceled and lateness to sessions than is seen with patients in private psychotherapy. Another serious outcome is the frequency with which patients' prematurely terminate their treatment, often without advance notice to the therapist. The average length of a managed care psychotherapy appears to be far shorter than the average duration of a private psychotherapy—a finding that does not preclude long-term treatment for some patients. Even so, the general thinness of patients' engagement in their therapy also make it far more difficult to involve them in generating the narrative material needed for, and doing their part of the work required by, psychodynamic and adaptive forms of treatment. There also is a tendency for some of these patients to blatantly resist accepting trigger decoded interpretation consciously even in the face of deep unconscious, encoded validation—detachment is served in this manner.

All in all, there are many factors that discourage managed care patients from making a full commitment to their therapists and therapies. These interfering pressures push these treatment situations towards fragmentation and create difficulties in achieving insightful symptom resolution, much to the disadvantage of both parties to the therapy—and their insurers as well. Here too, working with patients to enable them to gain deep insight into the sources of these problems and to begin to resolve their commitment issues is the best available ameliorative.

Therapists' Commitment to Treatment

I have already alluded to many factors that diminish the commitment of psychotherapists to their managed care patients and their psychotherapy. The above-mentioned fact that most patients select their therapist based on nothing more than their being on a list of providers diminishes the investment in treatment by the therapist as much as the patient. Therapists also react adversely to their patients' frequent latenesses and absences from sessions and to the loss of income that comes from advance-notice, non-payment cancellations and sudden terminations that are made without taking responsibility for the fee for the final scheduled session. These psychological wounds at the hands of managed care patient prompt many therapists to distance themselves protectively from all of their managed care clients.

Therapists also tend to be put off by their poorly committed patients' not uncommon requests for make-up sessions and for changes in the time of their appointments. The low fee that the therapist is paid for the treatment sessions and the small amount of a patient's co-pay also serve as restraints on therapists' full commitment to their patients. Delays in payments by patients or insurers and other fee issues that arise in connection with managed care treatment also have distancing effects. The managed care psychotherapy patient is an indiscriminating client who has no conscious means of differentiating sound from unsound therapists and therapies. As a result, the skills and healing powers of therapists who truly possess expertise often go unappreciated by both patients and insurers. This too contributes to the difficulties therapists have in making full commitments to their patients, a problem that is compounded by therapists' awareness that they can easily be replaced on a whim by their patients. Paradoxically, a therapist's awareness that for his or her part he or she can replace lost patients with relative ease keeps him or her from making the kind of investment in an ongoing therapy that is made with a private patient.

Still other distancing factors include a therapist's awareness that his or her work with patients is or may be under direct scrutiny by the insurer. The prospect of requests for process notes and other documentation related to the therapy with a given patient causes providers to experience insurers as intrusive, interfering, and relatively unsophisticated observers who create barriers that distant them from their patients. In addition, therapists often are concerned that an adverse turn in the course of a patient's psychotherapy could lead to a complaint to the insurer by the disillusioned patient. Another interfering factors lies with the sometimes explicit, but always implicit, pressures from insurers to comply with ill-defined so-called standard psychotherapy practices, even when the therapist is convinced that another approach to the therapy of a particular patient is called for; this too gives an impersonal cast to the therapeutic relationship. Similar consequences stem from the continuous pressures from some insurers that treatment be as brief as possible and that use be made of psychotropic medication—an innovation that may or may not support insight-oriented treatment, but all too often interferes with, and substitutes for, the mutual pursuit of deep understanding.

Along other lines, psychiatrists who see another therapist's patient for medication management and who do so in very brief sessions are likely to be relatively disinvested in the patient's care—a natural but unfortunate reaction that the psychiatrist should try to overcome. Then too, the oft-mentioned basic frame modifications of managed care psychotherapy also create barriers between therapists and their patients. All of this works against a strong therapeutic alliance between the parties to treatment. Barriers also stem from a therapist being required in many cases to obtain approval from the insurer for extensions of a patient's therapy; this loss of autonomy is a distancing factor for both parties to therapy. Additional detrimental factors include the fact that some patients do not have full coverage for the number of sessions ideally needed for them to gain symptom relief; pressures on the therapist to limit the frequency of sessions in many cases to once weekly; and the conscious and deep unconscious guilt that therapists experience over their having to violate the patient's right to full privacy and confidentiality.

In many cases, the practical consequences of these distancing conditions are a tendency in managed care therapists to be loose about giving their patients their full attention and therapeutic devotion and an inclination to be lax about managing the ground rules of treatment. This is especially true of their keeping to their responsibility to attend all scheduled sessions, to begin and end these hours on time, and to keep strict boundaries regarding self-revelations.

Finally, these interfering factors tend to cause a diminution of the compelling deep unconscious bond between the parties to therapy that accrues to secured-frame therapies. Such a bond strengthens the conscious therapeutic alliance, the emotional commitment to therapy by both patient and therapist, and the healing process itself. Distancing is intensified in managed care therapeutic relationships on both the conscious and deep unconscious levels of experience.

Once again we see how critical it is for therapists to be mindful of the conditions under which they work with managed care patients and the effects of these conditions on both their patients and themselves. Therapists are well advised to be aware of these issues and to find insightful ways to mobilize their commitment to their patients so as to fulfill all of their responsibilities as mental health professionals and healers. Engaging in self-processing and self-exploration, learning how to deal with and resolve many of the impediments to the deep unconscious intimacy and rapport needed for effective psychotherapy, and establishing a core of deep unconscious empathy with the patient should be major goals for all managed care psychotherapists.

THE FEASIBILITY OF SUCCESSFUL THERAPY

While statistical studies indicate that in general many forms of psychotherapy, cognitive and psychodynamic, are relatively successful undertakings, there are still a host of uncertainties and problems with these findings and with the effectiveness psychotherapy in general; they are yet to be effectively addressed. I shall therefore base my comments about the likelihood of symptom alleviation in managed care psychotherapy based on my accumulated impressions from doing and supervising managed care psychotherapy and from managing medications for patients in treatment with other therapists.

Overall, my experiences suggest that, as is true for psychotherapy at large, there is enormous variability in the care offered by psychotherapists to their managed care patients and in the outcome of these treatment experiences. I have seen in my own work and the work of others strikingly successful outcomes, but strikingly poor results as well. Clearly, there is much to mitigate against a sound cure for the patient, but most of these counter-therapeutic aspects of managed care therapy are primarily frame-related and they can be either overcome or partially resolved through interpretation and frame rectification efforts.

That said, I am nevertheless struck by the frequency with which managed care patients who are in psychotherapy with other therapists working under a variety of banners are referred to me for psychotropic medication. Consciously, most of these patients—and many of them have been in treatment for years—do not see the turn to pharmacological help as a reflection of problems in, or failures of, their psychotherapy; instead, they tend naively to accept this development as a turn to a supposedly minor supportive addendum. Indeed, adaptive studies indicate that patients' conscious evaluations of the status of their psychotherapies are quite unreliable and in most cases are skewed towards idealization far more than criticism, although with severely disruptive therapists, the latter does occur as well. Trigger decoding is necessary in order to ascertain the truth about a given therapy.

There is, then, an inordinate amount of denial operative in both patients and therapists in regard to the problems inherent to managed care treatment situations. This denial appears to have been especially strong in patients whom I medicated who were doing extremely poorly with their primary therapists—which is why they were referred to me for medication in the first place. These individuals showed symptomatic regressions and striking failures to improve clinically, and they tended to tell encoded stories that conveyed unconscious perceptions to the effect that they were not being helped by their therapists and in most cases, were experiencing considerable harm. Nevertheless, virtually always, they spoke consciously of the benefits of their sessions and the helpfulness of their therapists. Indeed, the evident denial reflected in these manifest statements are among the motives that prompted me to investigate the subject of love in psychotherapy (Langs 2006), only to discover that false forms of conscious love abound, especially in managed care treatment situations.

There are, then, serious limitations to the ability of conscious minds to fairly judge the status of a given psychotherapy experience. For unconscious reasons, therapists who avoid death and its encumbrances tend in general to be favored over those who pick up such themes and eventually interpret their sources and meanings. In addition, patients' deep unconscious guilt and needs for punishment for the harm they have caused others unwittingly motivate them to seek damaging rather than truly healing therapists. Such counter-therapeutic needs, which also are a factor in many forms of private therapy, are very common in managed care situations. As always, trigger decoding patients' deep unconscious perceptions of the quality of and underlying factors in a given treatment experience is the best way to ensure a favorable outcome to the therapy.

All in all, there is considerable need for fresh clinical research into the process and outcome of managed care psychotherapies. My overall impression is that even though there are extensive obstacles to cure, an effective healing process can take place under managed care conditions and a favorable result can be effected. I have seen it happen, but needless to say, much effort is required to achieve this goal.

ADAPTIVE PSYCHOTHERAPY REVISITED

I turn now to the particular difficulties that I have experienced in using the adaptive approach with managed care patients. Some of these problems apply to psychodynamic therapies in general and thus are of concern to all dynamically oriented psychotherapists. Others are specific to the adaptive approach, which is, as I said, centered on the process of trigger decoding as it illuminates the activated deep unconscious sources of patients' emotional distress, which is, at bottom, the result of death-related traumas and the death anxieties that they have engendered.

Clinical experience indicates that about one in four managed care patients to whom I suggest the adaptive form of narrative therapy accept my proposal and enter treatment. About half of these patients remain in therapy for an extended period of time, many of them one to three years. Those who do so tend, by and large, to be natural narrators who amply convey encoded deep unconscious memories and current experiences that facilitate unconsciously validated trigger decoded interpretations and frame-securing efforts, and by this means, gain notable symptom relief and improved functioning. Many of these patients are dealing with a repressed or obliterated significant early childhood trauma and they are able, in the course of the therapy and, to be sure, in the face of many resistances, to eventually either recover the trauma consciously or work it through based on encoded representations alone. Trigger decoded reconstructions usually play a significant role in this process.

This perspective may seem to be out of sync with the many pitfalls of managed care treatment to which I have previously alluded. But I have not identified these problems in order to malign or reject this type of psychotherapy. Instead, my intention has been to highlight the many generally unrecognized obstacles to cure—none of them necessarily fatal to a given treatment—so therapists and insurers can find ways to deal with and resolve as many of them as possible. Indeed, it is clear to me that much good is being done by psychotherapists working under the managed care banner. The unique problems raised by doing adaptive therapy with managed care patients tend to be quite similar to, and exaggerated versions of, those seen in private practice settings.

Patients' emotion-processing minds are adaptive entities that endeavor to cope, consciously and deep unconsciously, through both revelation and concealment, insight and defense, with the adaptation-evoking triggering events within and outside of therapy as they arise in the course of their therapeutic experiences. While the deviant managed care frame creates a bias toward concealment, revelations do transpire and therapeutic insight can be achieved. As noted, many moments in which a frame modification becomes an active issue can be turned to good stead when narrative material is generated by the patient and the therapist is able to offer unconsciously validated trigger decoded interpretations and frame rectifications where feasible. Such work offers patients much in the way of insightful emotional healing. Indeed, one favorable outcome is the weaning of many patients from psychotropic medications. Much of the success is founded on the adaptive principle of securing as much of the ground rules as possible. This effort provides patients with the safety and security, and deep unconscious emotional bond, they need to encode and eventually explore consciously their most severe traumas and death anxieties.

All in all, I have found this work to be both frustrating and deeply satisfying. It has given me an opportunity to work adaptively with a large number of patients who come from a wide variety of backgrounds and suffer from a wide range of emotional problems, psychotic and non-psychotic; for a psychoanalyst this is seldom the case. It also has enabled me to collect sufficient clinical data to confirm and, where needed, revise many aspects of the adaptive theoretical position and its enormous power to heal. It has been striking, for example, to see the consistency with which patients in their initial sessions consistently generate themes that, much to their conscious surprise and responsive denial, touch on the problems connected with the deviant conditions of managed care therapies such as the lack of total privacy and confidentiality. In addition, this work has presented me with lively new challenges, especially the need to search for fresh ways to help unconsciously terrified patients to remain in adaptive treatment and for patients of all kinds to benefit as much as possible from this form of therapy. As Freud said decades ago, therapists learn the most from cases that do not go well. Resistant managed care patients have compelled me to face and deal with the limitations of my knowledge base and healing powers, and have called on me to learn more and more about the emotion-processing mind and the effects of the ground rules of treatment on the therapeutic experience. Fittingly, these patients remind me again and again of the inevitable frustrations and difficulties of doing and being in psychotherapy—and in living our lives from day to day.

INSURER-RELATED FRAME ISSUES

Managed care psychotherapy involves three basic frames—one for the interactions between beneficiaries and insurers, another for the interplay between providers and insurers, and the third for the therapeutic interactions between therapist-providers and beneficiaries. These are, of course, inter-related frames and the ideals for each are based on universal frame-related archetypes even as each has its individual features—its own particular ground rules and boundaries. By and large, the handling of the frame of one of these interaction will influence the frames of, and parties to, the interactions within the other two frames. Because of this, everyone involved in managed care therapy needs to be mindful of the status of all three frameworks and of the nature and effects of frame-related interventions in each of them.

The final pathway in this complicated situation involves the patient and therapist and their therapeutic pursuits. For example, a fee dispute between a provider and an insurer—for example, a disagreement about the ground rule pertaining to patients' responsibility for fees for missed sessions—is likely to come to the attention of the patient and the outcome of the discussion most certainly will affect his or her view of the therapist and experience of the therapeutic frame. More dramatically, if an insurer fails to pay for a session or cancels the benefits of an insured, this frame-related action will have devastating effects on the patient, therapist, and treatment and it may lead to an abrupt termination of the therapy by the patient. In the extreme, should an insurer refuse or end benefits to a given patient and the patient is unable or refuses to pay the full fee for subsequent sessions (and it should be identical to that paid by the insurer), it may well be the therapist who terminates the treatment. This decision is an unusual way to secure the therapy frame in that it precludes seeing the patient at a reduced fee, yet it involves the end of the therapy. In these cases, it seems best to try to work out a compromised fee that is greater than the patient's copay and less than the total amount of money the therapist has been receiving from the patient's co-pay and the insurer's payments. This solution also is unusual in that it entails modifying the frame to secure the continuation of the treatment.

Insurers come into play largely around fee issues and decisions regarding extensions of an ongoing therapy. While I have heard many complaints about the ways in which insurers handle these issues, in relation to my own work this has seldom been a problem, much of it, I suspect, because I see all managed care therapy patients once weekly—the greater the frequency of sessions, the greater the chance of issues with the insurer.

Much of what happens regarding contested continuations of therapy depends on the action taken by the insurer and the rules that are stated in the contract between the patient and the insurer. If the insurer's decision to end coverage is in keeping with the contract, the patient and therapist may be upset, but they also have to recognize the legitimacy of the insurer's position. When patients' care is threatened, therapists still must maintain their neutrality in these situations and refrain from becoming third-party intruders into the insurer-patient frame and interaction. Therapists can be most helpful to their patients by continuing to hold the psychotherapy frame as steady as possible and by interpreting the relevant encoded themes in the patient's material as it comes up in the therapy.

Efforts by therapists to extend themselves in order to rescue the patient vis-à-vis the insurer or to offer unconsciously damaging frame violations to the patient are to be avoided. On the other hand, if need be and can be honestly stated, it is incumbent on the therapist to provide the patient and insurer with a report that indicates why the coverage and sessions should be continued. The therapist does, however, become the patient's advocate, thereby abandoning his or her neutrality—a frame deviation that needs to be interpreted and rectified based on trigger decoding the patient's responsive imagery. Still, the ultimate power in these matters usually resides with the insurer, a fact that affects both the patient and therapist. All of these frame-related entanglements need to be processed with the patient as his or her narrative communications allow. In the end, if the insurer will not support further sessions, the therapist, as noted, should try to find a basis for continuing the patient's therapy on a private basis, usually by offering to charge the patient a reasonable fee that he or she can afford.

Managed care psychotherapists often have their own frame issues with the insurers with whom they have contracted. Therapists may be asked for superfluous information about their patients and may have their overall work with patients reviewed by insurers from time to time. The models of treatment used in these evaluations do, however, tend to be rigid, ill-informed dynamically, and thus a poor basis for criticizing a skillful insight-oriented therapist's work. Issues with insurers also may arise in regard to continuing therapy with a given patient, as may problems related to fees, the specific medications a psychiatrist prescribes, and similar matters. Therapists' conscious and unconscious reactions to these intrusions will affect their therapeutic efforts with their patients, so they need to be mindful of the multi-level effects of these sometimes necessary, and at times unnecessary, frame modifications. Whatever their nature—and they need to be shared by the therapist with the patient—the effects of these frame-related transactions on the therapist-insurer relationship strongly influence the transactions between the patient and therapist. At times, effects may transpire in the reverse direction in that transactions within the psychotherapy may have a profound effect on an insurer's decisions regarding the patient, therapist, and the psychotherapy. Much damage can be done unless these matters are handled properly by the therapist and the conscious and deep unconscious effects on the patient worked through and if possible, resolved.

Let the buyer and provider of managed care services beware: A third party holds much of the power as overseers of their therapeutic efforts. This often frustrating higher power must be dealt with without undue rancor and at all times, with the best interests of the patient as the paramount commitment.

Chapter Nine

Three Sets of Recommendations

I shall conclude this exploration of managed care psychotherapy with a series of recommendations to each of the three parties involved in this process—insurers, providers, and beneficiaries. The goals of these recommendations are straightforward:

To foster the development of educational programs for all three parties to the managed care situation.

To improve the care offered by managed care mental health providers.

To reduce the overall cost of mental health care for both insurers and beneficiaries.

To improve the fees paid to providers.

To lessen the length of time needed to achieve symptom relief in a managed care treatment experience.

To eliminate the inclination of providers and beneficiaries to engage in fraudulent billing practices and other illegal or inappropriate measures in their dealings with each other and with their insurers.

To facilitate the offer by managed care therapists of the best possible, healing, supportive therapeutic environment for the therapy of the patient.

To improve the relationships and cooperation between the three parties to managed care psychotherapy.

To make working in a managed care setting a largely gratifying experience for both psychotherapists and their patients.

To render the outcome of the treatment process as favorable as possible.

INSURERS

Insurers need to have a core group of informed managers for the field of mental health. They in turn should make efforts to acquire a deep understanding of the emotion-processing mind and its responses to the managed care therapeutic environment so they may regulate in keeping with the special needs of the field. To do so, they also need to comprehend the nature of psychodynamic forms of treatment in order to better appreciate the intricacies of the therapeutic environment and the treatment experience. They need, then, to be frame-sensitive and to appreciate the multiple effects, conscious and deeply unconscious, of the framework of managed care treatments. And they should do so despite the fact that most of their contracted therapists do not appreciate the importance of these highly critical frame issues. They also will need to engage in the difficult task of defining broadly the features of sound and unsound therapeutic practices as derived from the various schools of psychotherapy. They need to become informed overseers. Achieving this kind of fresh understanding should lead insurers to refashion and revise aspects of their managed care contracts with both their insured and their providers so that the needs of all concerned are better met in ways that favorably influence the healing of the insured and yet are cost effective as well.

Insurers also should make stronger efforts to communicate with and educate their mental health providers and beneficiaries—current programs are infrequent, often poorly timed to conflict with therapists' working hours, and too narrowly focused to be of help to most therapists. Insurance companies also need to develop viable vehicles for sustaining these contacts. The goal should be to teach and support sound therapeutic efforts and to cooperatively effect constructive changes in the basic managed care contract and its prescribed ground rules. Toward these ends, insurers are well advised to arrange for the distribution of books on psychotherapy and related subjects that have been carefully screened by panels of experts for the viability and the validity of their points of view. Insurers also should sponsor more seminars, lectures, on-line chat groups, and research studies pertaining to the managed care frame and other aspects of the managed care treatment experience and its outcome. The use of questionnaires sent to both providers and the insured seems advisable.

Most importantly, insurers need to form committees of therapists who are sophisticated in regard to ground rule and frame issues and the therapeutic process. They should then ask these individuals to review existing managed care contracts with an eye toward recommending advantageous changes that include securing those deviant ground rules that are open to such measures. High on this list should be a reconsideration of the prevailing policy of allowing patients who give advance notice to their therapists to forgo responsibility for payment of the therapist's fee for that session. This ground rule undermines the effectiveness of the therapy; promotes anti-therapeutic recidivism in patients and their pathological use of frame deviations in both the treatment setting and everyday life; creates unnecessary financial hardships for managed care therapists; and may well be costing insurers millions of dollars each year in unjustified and erroneously rationalized false billing practices.

The best way to resolve this problem appears to be a shift in policy to holding patients who are being seen in regularly scheduled sessions responsible for the full fee for all missed sessions regardless of the cause. A possible but less viable compromise would be to mandate that patients pay the co-pay for all missed sessions, but this is an unnecessary concession to the frame-deviant needs of all concerned. The practical problem with this last suggestion is that many patients cancel sessions for frivolous reasons and insurers need to create an all-embracing ground rule that does not ask therapists' to judge the validity of a patient's reason for missing a session. While the change to patients' full responsibility for canceled sessions is a way that insurers can show their respect and concern for their providers, it also is a way that insurers show their respect and concern for their insured—they too will benefit emotionally from a ground rule of this kind. Insurers should make this responsibility clear to their clients, explain its necessity, and indicate that it pertains to consultation sessions as well as to sessions that are part of an ongoing therapy experience. Thus, insurers need to make special efforts to inform potential patients that therapists work with scheduled hours that cannot be filled once a commitment is made and that they must accept the responsibility to be present for all arranged hours, including the initial visit. This touches on the much-neglected need for insurers to better educate their insured regarding the many facets of the psychotherapy process—efforts that must, however, be well informed and deeply insightful.

Also in need of correction is the practice of some insurers to offer fees for psychotherapy sessions with medication management that are higher than those for psychotherapy alone. This imbalance encourages medical therapists to prescribe psychotropic drugs for patients for whom their use is marginal or uncalled-for. It also opens the door to deceitful billing practices. This arrangement is patently unfair to non-medical therapists and to medical therapists who choose to work with their patients using psychotherapy alone. It seems advisable for insurers to forgo this practice.

Much the same applies to the unjustifiable custom of some insurers to have pay scales that depend on the professional degree held by a provider and in some cases to pay higher fees to out-of-network providers than they do to those who are in-network—an arrangement that penalizes in-network therapists and is quite unjustified. Along similar lines, the practice of some insurers to use different fee scales for services rendered in different parts of the country also needs to be reconsidered. These inequities create resentment in providers and are among the sources of the conflicts that arise between insurers and providers, and between providers and their patients.

Another practice that is in need of reconsideration is the requirement by some insurers that their therapists routinely request authorization for such matters as initial consultations, the continuation of therapy beyond a fixed number of sessions, or the extension of treatment beyond the number of initially authorized sessions. With the possible exception of unusually long or intensive therapies, it seems advisable to allow patients and their therapists to determine if the patient is in need of ongoing therapy and how long the treatment should last.

Yet another recommendation calls for the creation of ombudsmen or liaisons between insurers and providers, and insurers and their beneficiaries. These individuals would deal mainly with problems that touch on matters of principle, but there also should be a means of considering individual complaints as well. The details of this recommendation should be worked out by teams of insurers, providers, and beneficiaries; putting this plan in place promises to greatly improve the atmosphere and working conditions of managed care treatment—and its therapeutic potential.

Finally, the fee scale for mental health professionals needs to be re-evaluated and a universal fee agreed on by the industry—providers are forbidden by law to bargain with individual insurers. The low fees paid to providers are demeaning and exploitative; they need to be increased and cost of living increases should be provided on a yearly basis. This aspect of the situation has been greatly aggravated by the availability of information about the corporate earnings of major insurers and the high individual earnings of their executives. This is not to question the salaries to which they are entitled, but to point out that the high salaries of some in-house staff contrasts with the low payments made to providers, a situation that has caused all manner of problems that damage all concerned.

PROVIDERS

As for providers, it is vital that they be open to new ideas relevant to the practice of psychotherapy regardless of their present clinical orientation. Basic topics like the evolution, design, and operations of the emotion-processing mind deserve their consideration, as does the basic role of unconscious processes in emotional health, its ills, and its psychotherapy. There also is an evident need for therapists to more fully grasp the critical role played by rules, frames, and boundaries in managed care psychotherapy, including the effects of the mandated frame modifications inherent to managed care treatment. These educational efforts are needed to widen the purview of managed care therapists regardless of their basic orientation and to thereby enhance their understanding of the human mind and the ins and outs of managed care treatments.

Therapists especially need to appreciate and understand the relationship between their management of the ground rules of managed care therapy and their ethical and moral positions vis-à-vis their patients. They also need to find ways to recognize the often dire consequences of unneeded frame violations and the salutary effects of frame securing efforts. There is as well an urgent need for therapists to fully comprehend the severely negative impact of deceitful billing and other deviant practices on both themselves and their patients.

All in all, there is a great deal of critical information about the therapeutic process and interaction that has not reached and been appreciated by most providers. The approach to psychotherapy and model of the mind with which they choose to work must, of course, be a matter of their own selection. But nevertheless, they should be open to learning as much as they can about the deep unconscious transactions and intricacies of the therapeutic experience and the influence of their interventions, frame-related and otherwise, so they can improve their work and therapeutic results with their patients and find greater satisfaction in these endeavors.

Fashioning a less naïve, educated class of providers is one way to enhance the rewards of managed care psychotherapy for themselves and their beleaguered clients.

BENEFICIARIES

Patients also will benefit from the offer of fresh educational materials and lectures. They too need to deeply understand the role played by the ground rules of managed care psychotherapy in their search for emotional relief. They therefore need to be informed about the workings of the emotion-processing mind; the role played by rules, frames, and boundaries in the therapeutic process; the features of sound psychotherapy; and the risks of poorly conducted treatment experiences. They also need to be informed about the existence of an ideal, archetypal psychotherapy frame, the consequences of departures from this optimal frame, and the ethical and deep unconscious consequences of their therapists' and their own attempts to modify the secured aspects of the conditions of their therapies. In addition, whatever the risks of abuse, patients need to have a sympathetic ear to which they can voice their complaints. This should also have a favorable effect on their approach to treatment and should improve their relationship with both their providers and their insurers.

CONCLUDING COMMENTS

My extended exploration of managed care psychotherapy and medication management has been fashioned mainly to identify and offer possible solutions to largely overlooked issues and to issues that are well known but have heretofore eluded resolution. The over-riding focus has been on the ground rules and framework of managed care therapy, their nature, and influence—a focus that stems from the fundamental effects that the frame has on every aspect of managed care therapy, including its outcome. Managed care psychotherapy brings the much-neglected role and effects of therapists' frame management efforts into bold relief as the backbone of the psychotherapy experience. In brief, neglect the frame and you neglect the heart of the psychotherapy experience; honor the frame and you will have an honorable and healing psychotherapy experience.

All in all, my hope is that I have given readers, be they managed care patients, providers, or insurers, fresh perspectives and critical insights into the many often daunting problems that accrue to this mode of treatment, along with clues as how they can best be dealt with and resolved to the greatest extent feasible. In the emotional realm, being realistic about the role of reality in emotional life and the therapeutic process and understanding its influence in depth are vital to being able to negotiate the most favorable resolutions to the inevitable problems that realities, past and present, within and outside of therapy, present to us.

Therapists and insurers, and properly educated recipients of care, need to work to implement the many changes that can favorably affect the managed care psychotherapy experience. As is the case with our understanding of the emotion-processing mind and emotional life, this kind of work is never finished, but sound efforts to advance our insights and the clinical skills of practicing therapists can take us another step forward in our pursuit of the ideal healing experience. It is my hope that this book will be seen as one of these advances that are so sorely needed in the managed care scene.

Bibliography

Freud, S. *The Interpretation of Dreams*. Standard Edition 4 and 5, 1900.

Jung, C. "Analytic Psychology: Its Theory and Practice." In *The Tavistock Lectures*. London: Routledge & Kegan Paul, 1968.

Langs, R. *Madness and Cure*. Lake Worth, Fl: Gardner Press, 1985.

——. *Empowered Psychotherapy*. London: Karnac Books, 1993.

——. *Death Anxiety in Clinical Practice*. London: Karnac Books, 1997.

——. *Ground Rules in Psychotherapy and Counselling*. London: Karnac Books, 1998.

——. *Fundamentals of Adaptive Psychotherapy and Counselling*. London: Palgrave-Macmillan, 2004.

——. *Love and Death in Psychotherapy*. London: Palgrave-Macmillan, 2006.

——. *Beyond Yahweh and Jesus: Bringing Death's Wisdom to Faith, Spirituality, and Psychoanalysis*. Lanham, Md: Jason Aronson, 2008.

Index